The
Science
of
Nutrition

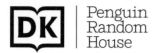

Art Editor Alison Gardner
Editors Andrea Page, Holly Kyte, Salima Hirani
Project Designer Louise Brigenshaw
Senior Editor Alastair Laing
US Editor Jennette ElNaggar
Design Manager Marianne Markham
Managing Editor Dawn Henderson
DTP and Design Coordinator Heather Blagden
Production Editor David Almond
Production Controller Luca Bazzoli
Jacket Coordinator Lucy Philpott
Art Director Maxine Pedliham
Publishing Director Katie Cowan

Photographer Stephanie McLeod
Illustrators Nelli Velichko, Sally Caulwell

First American Edition, 2021
Published in the United States by DK Publishing
1450 Broadway, Suite 801, New York, NY 10018

A catalog record for this book
is available from the Library of Congress.
ISBN 978-0-7440-3989-4

Printed and bound in China

For the curious
www.dk.com

RHIANNON LAMBERT

The Science of Nutrition

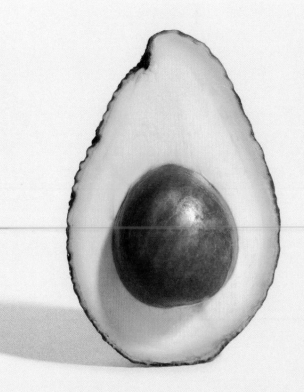

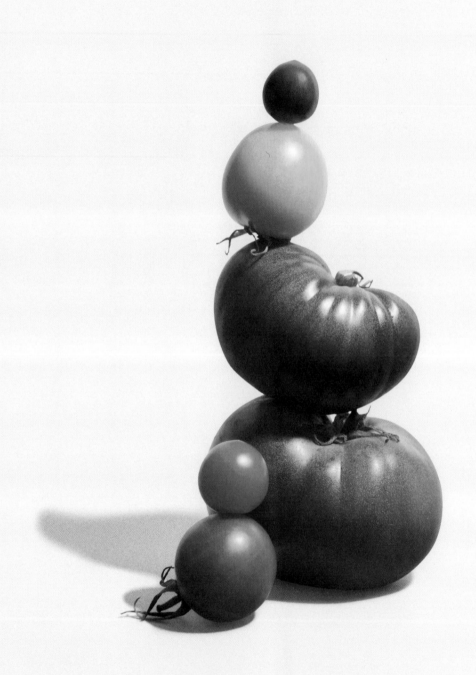

CONTENTS

INTRODUCTION

Enrolling to study nutrition at the University of Roehampton was a life-changing decision for me. It was one that, in part, I was driven to from firsthand experience of how easily we can fall into dysfunctional relationships with food, how pressures to look a certain way can lead to a pursuit of dietary quick fixes that are a world away from a relaxed and healthy enjoyment of food.

At the age of 17, I was an aspiring soprano singer, thrust into the limelight having won Classic FM's young musician of the year. Schooled at The Royal Academy of Music and singing on stage at the likes of the Royal Albert Hall and Paris Fashion Week, I appeared to be living the most thrilling life.

But after four years suffering the pressures of the music industry, compounded by fueling myself with passing dietary fads, I looked at my career and thought, I don't want this anymore. While a complete career change is rare, it is one of the best moves I ever made.

Following four grueling yet thrilling years, I obtained undergraduate and master's degrees in nutrition and started a new life as a fledgling nutritionist. Having founded Rhitrition in 2016, a private Harley Street clinic, my specialist team and I now work with individuals and leading brands to support their health and well-being. Our ethos is simply that we believe in empowering everyone to embrace a healthy way of living through the food we enjoy and the life we lead. Our bodies are as unique as our personalities, so each of us should strive to find a way of eating that works for us individually.

It is through my experience in clinic that I have come to learn just how widespread pseudoscience is. It's everywhere, from the labels in the supermarket, on the ads that pop up in your Instagram feed, and most of all in magazines—bold statements in jargon that give the false impression they're supported by laboratory research. With this book, I'm betting on the opposite approach—cold, hard facts that will teach you and help shape the way you think about food like never before.

Covering every conceivable topic—from gut bacteria to weight management to heart health and immune support to vegan diets and intermittent fasting (and everything in between)—*The Science of Nutrition* offers clear answers with informative graphics, making it easy to understand. I know that in debunking popular myths and diets, this book will enable you to make informed decisions that are best suited to you, about what, when, and how to eat responsibly for health and happiness.

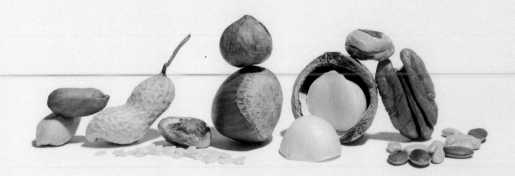

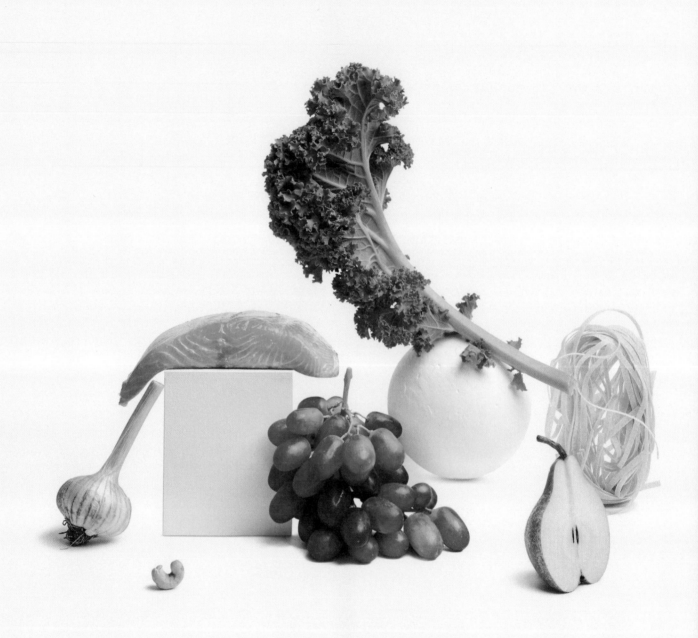

WHAT IS NUTRITION?

WHAT DO WE MEAN BY NUTRITION?

Nutrition is the process by which we provide the body with the nutrients necessary for good health and growth. Essentially, nutrition is nourishment for the body via the foods you eat.

Eating nutritiously enables you to enjoy the sense of well-being that comes with good health. Adequate nutrition is vital if you want your body to be healthy and well maintained and have the best chance at fighting disease and operating optimally.

We get our nourishment mostly from macronutrients, which are the dietary main players, but micronutrients are no less important. A balanced diet contains many different types of both.

MACRONUTRIENTS

There are three macronutrients: carbohydrates (see pages 12–13), protein (see pages 14–15), and fat (see pages 16–17). These three macronutrients give your body the energy it needs to operate.

The body takes care of many processes that require energy without our conscious control (such as breathing, temperature regulation, digestion, and cell repair). And, of course, your body requires energy for movement. Each of the macronutrients is required in relatively large amounts every day to support many of your body's vital functions.

MICRONUTRIENTS

We need vitamins and minerals, known as micronutrients, in much smaller quantities than macronutrients, but they are vital for the body to carry out its functions. In children, they are also essential for healthy growth and development.

Because we need macronutrients in much larger quantities than micronutrients, it's easy to underestimate the importance of the latter and focus more on including the former in the diet. But the absence of micronutrients can lead to severe consequences. The World Health Organization suggests that micronutrient deficiency is responsible for some of the most common nutritional deficiencies, such as anemia (iron), rickets, and osteoporosis (vitamin D), all of which can have a debilitating effect on the body's well-being and performance.

You can get most of your vitamins and minerals from plants. Plant foods come in various colors and shades, and their color is linked to the nutrients they contain. For instance, orange often indicates the presence of vitamin A; purples indicate antioxidants; greens contain vitamin K and iron; and red vegetables contain lots of vitamin C. So a colorful diet will give you a well-varied nutrient intake.

The daily requirement of each micronutrient varies between individuals, but if your diet is healthy and balanced, including foods from both plants and animal sources, you are likely to be ingesting all the micronutrients your body needs without the need for supplements. For those who don't eat animal products, a well-thought-through diet alongside targeted supplementation will provide the essential nutrients you need (see pages 128–131). However, do see a registered dietitian nutritionist if you want to enhance your diet for optimal performance.

Unique nutritional needs

THERE IS NO ONE-SIZE-FITS-ALL IN NUTRITION.
Your optimal intake of each macronutrient and
micronutrient depends on numerous factors. Your age,
gender, genetics, metabolism, level of physical activity,
and personal preferences all have a part to play in
establishing the best foods to keep working optimally.
Learn to listen to your body and notice how you feel
in response to your diet. See your primary care
physician if at all concerned.

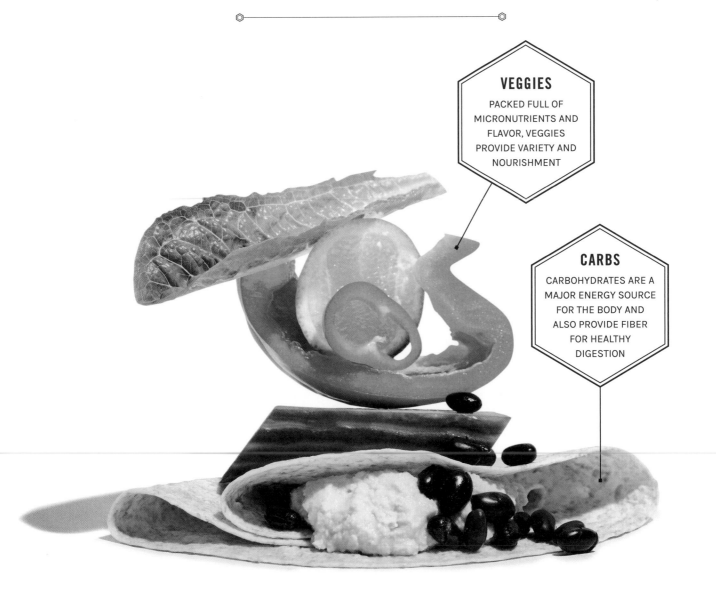

VEGGIES
PACKED FULL OF
MICRONUTRIENTS AND
FLAVOR, VEGGIES
PROVIDE VARIETY AND
NOURISHMENT

CARBS
CARBOHYDRATES ARE A
MAJOR ENERGY SOURCE
FOR THE BODY AND
ALSO PROVIDE FIBER
FOR HEALTHY
DIGESTION

WHAT ARE CARBOHYDRATES?

Carbohydrates are the body's greatest energy source. They provide the body with glucose to use for energy, which can also be stored (as glycogen) for future use. Carbs also play a valuable role in gut health, by providing useful fiber to the digestive tract.

Glucose is the preferred energy source for muscles during strenuous exercise. It is only when the body's glucose supply is depleted that it turns to fat for energy. The body also requires glucose to fuel multiple unconscious biological processes.

Glucose is essential fuel for the brain, aiding in concentration. Carbohydrates play an important role in generating the brain's serotonin supply. This mood-regulating hormone is made with tryptophan, an amino acid (see page 15) obtained through protein in the diet. Carbs help convert tryptophan into serotonin, so eating carbs may help enhance mood. This might explain why carbs and sweet foods are often treated as comfort foods.

There isn't enough research to show that consuming higher quantities of carbs or protein-rich foods containing tryptophan supports mood improvement in humans. However, it may be the case that low-carb consumption causes low mood.

If you've ever been on a diet that involves avoiding carbs, you may have experienced mood swings and found it hard to concentrate. You may have also felt fatigued. Serotonin is converted to melatonin, a hormone that helps regulate circadian rhythm.

DIGESTING CARBS

In the small intestine (see page 28), the less starchy complex carbs are broken down into simple carbs (see below). All non-glucose monosaccharides are converted into glucose in the liver, which is released

---

Simple and complex carbs

Monosaccharides (sugar in its simplest molecular form) and disaccharides are simple carbohydrates. Complex carbs comprise many monosaccharides and also contain starch in varying levels. Less starchy complex carbs include broccoli, zucchini, tomato, and eggplant. Examples of starchier complex carbs are potatoes, beans, and corn.

SINGLE MOLECULE

Monosaccharides
"Mono" means "one"; "saccharide" means "sugar." These are carbs in their most basic form.

GLUCOSE
grains, pasta

FRUCTOSE
fruit, honey

GALACTOSE
dairy

TWO MOLECULES

Disaccharides
When two monosaccharides bond chemically, they form a disaccharide.

LACTOSE
DAIRY

SUCROSE
sugar beet, cane sugar

MALTOSE
molasses, beer

MULTIPLE MOLECULES

Polysaccharide
Carbs can be made up of hundreds, even thousands, of monosaccharides. These are called complex carbs.

many vegetables, beans, lentils, and whole grains

into the bloodstream. It is either used immediately or converted into glycogen (a polysaccharide of glucose), which is stored in the liver and muscles for later use (see pages 110–111).

Fiber (see pages 18–19) refers to any complex carbohydrates that cannot be broken down by the digestive enzymes in the small intestine (see pages 28–29). This fibrous matter moves into the large intestine, where it helps produce highly useful short-chain fatty acids and nourishes the lining of the gut.

"GOOD" AND "BAD" CARBS

There is no such thing as an inherently good or bad carb. All foods have a place—it's about finding the right balance for your own body. As a general rule, carbohydrates in their natural, fiber-rich form are more nutritious than those that have been stripped of their fiber content. Fruits and vegetables are excellent sources of carbohydrates.

There's a strong case for reducing refined carbs, like white bread, and opting for complex carbs, like whole grains (see p.45), which release energy slowly. While refined carbs are great for providing energy quickly, they usually lack essential nutrients. Many grain-based processed foods in the US are fortified or enriched with vitamins and minerals.

What does GI mean?

GLUCOSE FROM SIMPLE CARBS IS ABSORBED INTO THE BLOODSTREAM QUICKLY, WHILE COMPLEX CARBS TAKE LONGER TO BREAK DOWN. Glycemic index (GI) is a measure of how quickly a carbohydrate food will make your blood glucose levels rise after ingesting it. The higher the GI, the faster the impact. Glycemic load (GL) is a slightly different unit of measurement. It takes into account both the GI and the amount of carbohydrate in the food. So pasta has a lower GI than watermelon, yet pasta has more carbs and, therefore, a higher GL. If you eat similar amounts of both, the pasta will have the greater effect on your blood sugar levels.

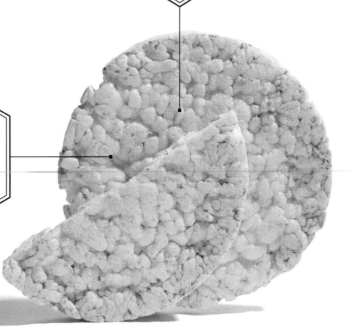

QUICK ENERGY

CONSISTING MOSTLY OF WHITE RICE AND AIR, RICE CAKES PROVIDE A LITTLE BIT OF ENERGY QUICKLY

NUTRIENT-LITE

FOR A MORE NUTRIENT-RICH OPTION, CHOOSE BROWN RICE CAKES OR WHOLE GRAIN CRACKERS

Rice cakes Many people presume these popular low-calorie snacks are healthy when, in fact, they are also low in nutrients.

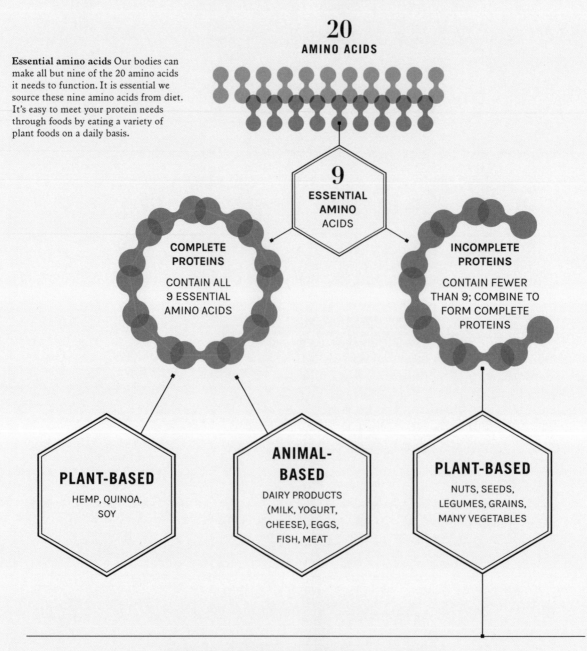

20
AMINO ACIDS

Essential amino acids Our bodies can make all but nine of the 20 amino acids it needs to function. It is essential we source these nine amino acids from diet. It's easy to meet your protein needs through foods by eating a variety of plant foods on a daily basis.

9
ESSENTIAL
AMINO
ACIDS

COMPLETE PROTEINS
CONTAIN ALL 9 ESSENTIAL AMINO ACIDS

INCOMPLETE PROTEINS
CONTAIN FEWER THAN 9; COMBINE TO FORM COMPLETE PROTEINS

PLANT-BASED
HEMP, QUINOA, SOY

ANIMAL-BASED
DAIRY PRODUCTS (MILK, YOGURT, CHEESE), EGGS, FISH, MEAT

PLANT-BASED
NUTS, SEEDS, LEGUMES, GRAINS, MANY VEGETABLES

POPULAR PAIRINGS OF INCOMPLETE PROTEINS:

LENTILS + RICE

OATS + NUTS

BROWN RICE + BLACK BEANS

PEANUT BUTTER + WHOLE GRAIN BREAD

HUMMUS + BREAD OR CRACKERS

BAKED BEANS ON WHOLE GRAIN TOAST

NOODLES IN A PEANUT SAUCE

BEAN BURGERS ON A BUN

LENTILS OR BEANS WITH PASTA

WHAT IS PROTEIN?

The macronutrient protein is a major player in the diet. It is the body's building block, used to form and repair muscles, skin, hair, and nails, for instance. Protein also enables many of the body's vital metabolic functions.

Every single cell in the body contains protein, and there are thousands of types found in the body. Proteins form the structure of tissues. They also carry molecules around the body to where they are needed, playing an important role in many chemical reactions that take place, including immune response and the production and deployment of hormones.

Proteins are made up of amino acids. Short chains of amino acids are called peptides (they connect to each other with peptide bonds) while longer chains are called polypeptides or proteins. Protein chains can become complex in structure as more and more chains join and fold in on themselves. The body breaks down protein chains into peptides to use for specific purposes as required. For instance, the hormone insulin (see pages 172–173) is a peptide.

The body can produce many of the amino acids it needs to make peptides and proteins, but nine of them, known as essential amino acids, must be sourced from the diet (see opposite). Because the body doesn't store proteins in the same way it does other macronutrients, it needs to consume proteins every day. Numerous studies demonstrate that a diet with adequate protein has major health benefits.

FOOD SOURCES

Food sources containing all nine essential amino acids in sufficient quantities are known as complete proteins. They are found in animal products and a few plant sources.

Incomplete proteins are plant-based sources of protein that don't contain all nine essential amino acids, or don't have sufficient quantities of them to meet the body's daily requirements. Although "incomplete," they are no less valuable than complete proteins as protein needs are met across the whole day, not just at each individual meal.

Vegans and vegetarians are advised to eat a wide variety of protein-rich and fortified foods to ensure they consume all nine of the essential amino acids each day from both complete and incomplete sources (see pages 128–129).

PROTEIN INTAKE

Scientists agree that age, gender, and level of physical activity all determine how much protein to consume. In the US, adults are advised to consume 0.8g protein per kg (2lb) of bodyweight per day. (Particularly active people should increase this intake to 1g.) Based on average weights and activity levels, daily intake should be 56g for men and 46g for women. That's about two palm-size portions of meat, fish, tofu, nuts, or beans. Elderly people need up to 50 percent more than the recommended daily intake. As we grow older, our bodies become less efficient at using protein. Increasing protein intake makes it more likely we'll meet daily requirements.

I advise my clients to get as many complete protein sources in as possible throughout the day and/or focus on consuming a wide variety of incomplete sources.

When choosing what protein to eat, ensure the foods you pick give you the best all-around nutrition possible. Consider what other nutrients you are receiving with your protein sources.

And don't worry about getting everything in at one sitting—your protein input can add up throughout the day.

WHAT IS FAT?

Fat is a macronutrient found in many food sources. Consuming fats is vital to the body's function, including processes such as brain activity, hormone production, and the body's absorption of other nutrients from the diet.

We should aim to get one-third of our calories from fat. The fat we eat is broken down into triglycerides (fatty acid cells combined with glycerol, a type of glucose) that travel in the blood to wherever they will be used or stored.

There are two main types of dietary fats: saturated and unsaturated. Unsaturated fats are either monounsaturated or polyunsaturated. Most foods containing fat naturally contain a mixture of different types of fats, so it's difficult to exclude one type in favor of another. However, we should aim to cut down on saturated fats and opt for more monounsaturated and polyunsaturated fats.

Avoid the artificial additive transfat (see pages 58–59) due to its links to inflammation, unhealthy cholesterol levels, impaired artery function, insulin resistance (see page 172).

MONOUNSATURATED FATS

This type of unsaturated fat contains only one double bond in its molecular structure. Monounsaturated fats are linked to several health benefits, including a reduced risk of serious diseases such as heart disease and diabetes.

Monounsaturated fatty acids (MUFAs) are typically liquid at room temperature and are fairly stable for cooking purposes (see pages 66–67). The most common MUFA is oleic acid, which is present in olive oil in high amounts. Excellent sources of this healthy fat are avocados, nuts, seeds, canola oil, fish oils, and nut oils.

POLYUNSATURATED FATS

This type of unsaturated fat contains two or more double bonds in its structure. Polyunsaturated fatty acids (PUFAs) are found in sunflower seeds, oily fish, walnuts, flaxseeds, and vegetable oils, including safflower, sunflower, and corn oils.

Omega-3 and omega-6 are polyunsaturated fats. Omega-3 plays a crucial role in the production of hormones, in the immune system, blood clotting, and cellular growth. Studies show that consuming omega-3 fats is linked to reduced incidence of health conditions, including neurodegenerative disease, heart disease, and diabetes. We need to consider increasing our intake of omega-3 fats, as these are usually eaten in small quantities and found in less commonly consumed foods, like oily fish, flaxseeds, or walnuts.

SATURATED FATS

These come mainly from animal sources and tend to be solid at room temperature. Saturated fats are very stable at high temperatures and therefore less likely to be damaged during cooking. That's why, for instance, butter is used traditionally for baking cakes. Milk, cheese, fatty meats such as lamb, processed meat (sausages, burgers, and bacon), coconut oil, cakes, and cookies are sources of saturated fats.

While saturated fat plays a part in nutrition, too much in the diet is linked to heart disease. We still eat too much saturated fat in the US. No more than 5–6 percent of our total intake of calories should come from saturated fats.

Cholesterol

Cholesterol is a lipid (fatty substance) the body uses to build cells, among other things. Some cholesterol is obtained from diet, but much of the body's supply is made in the liver. It attaches to a protein to form tiny spheres (lipoproteins) that are carried in blood to wherever they are needed. There are two types: HDL and LDL.

HDL

High-density lipoproteins (HDL) are good cholesterol. These particles contain a high proportion of protein to cholesterol. They protect the body by carrying LDL cholesterol away from arteries to the liver, and they have anti-inflammatory properties.

LDL

Low-density lipoproteins (LDL) are bad cholesterol. They have a lower proportion of protein to cholesterol. These types of fatty acids carry cholesterol to the cells. Too much LDL can be harmful because it sticks to the inside walls of your arteries, causing buildup of fatty material, limiting blood flow and leading to heart conditions and stroke.

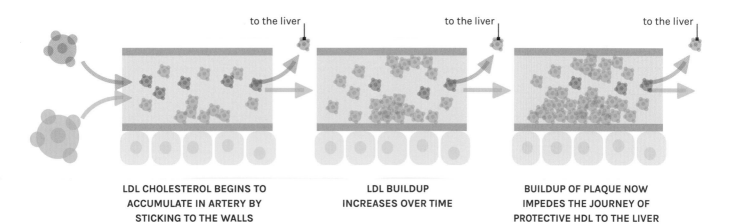

to the liver

LDL CHOLESTEROL BEGINS TO ACCUMULATE IN ARTERY BY STICKING TO THE WALLS

LDL BUILDUP INCREASES OVER TIME

BUILDUP OF PLAQUE NOW IMPEDES THE JOURNEY OF PROTECTIVE HDL TO THE LIVER

Increasing HDL and reducing LDL cholesterol

We want to aim for a preferential ratio between HDL and LDL cholesterol. There are measures we can take to increase our HDL cholesterol levels and lower LDL. Nondietary actions include exercising regularly and stopping smoking. Avoid transfats completely, and include the following foods regularly in your diet.

Purple fruits and vegetables are rich in anthocyanins, which may help increase HDL cholesterol levels.

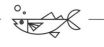

Oily fish 1-2 times a week may help increase HDL cholesterol levels and benefit heart health.

Olive oil increases HDL levels in healthy people, the elderly, and those with high LDL cholesterol.

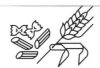

Whole grains are linked to a lower risk of heart disease. Oats and barley contain beta-glucan, which lowers LDL cholesterol.

Nuts are rich in cholesterol-lowering fats and fiber, as well as minerals that are linked to improved heart health.

Avocados contain monounsaturated fatty acids and fiber, both of which lower LDL cholesterol.

Legumes such as beans, peas, and lentils help lower LDL levels and are a good source of plant-based proteins.

WHAT IS FIBER?

Fiber is in part made of long chains of glucose molecules (polysaccharides, see pages 12–13). The small intestine is unable to break down the fiber content of carbs we consume. Fiber's passage through the digestive system is very beneficial for health.

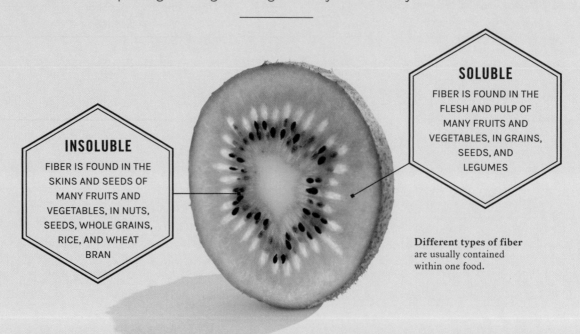

INSOLUBLE
FIBER IS FOUND IN THE SKINS AND SEEDS OF MANY FRUITS AND VEGETABLES, IN NUTS, SEEDS, WHOLE GRAINS, RICE, AND WHEAT BRAN

SOLUBLE
FIBER IS FOUND IN THE FLESH AND PULP OF MANY FRUITS AND VEGETABLES, IN GRAINS, SEEDS, AND LEGUMES

Different types of fiber are usually contained within one food.

Fiber keeps the digestive system healthy and in good working order. It slows down digestion, which regulates blood sugar levels, and helps us feel fuller longer, reducing the likelihood of weight gain. Most people don't eat enough of it, despite the positive health outcomes associated with consuming more of it. For each 8g increase in daily intake, we reduce the risk of type 2 diabetes by 15 percent, heart disease by 19 percent, and colon cancer by 80 percent.

SOLUBLE FIBER

This type of fiber dissolves in water to form a gel-like substance that helps make stools soft. This enables them to progress through the gut with ease, preventing constipation. Soluble fiber (in oats, for instance) slows down digestion, which helps with satiety (see page 104) and also with regulating blood sugar levels. Soluble fiber

has another great benefit; in the small intestine, its presence reduces the absorption of cholesterol into the bloodstream, which has the positive effect of reducing the levels of LDL cholesterol (the bad type of cholesterol; p.17) circulating in the blood.

INSOLUBLE FIBER

As the name suggests, insoluble fiber does not dissolve in water, so it can be only partially broken down by digestion. It helps to push things along in your digestive tract, preventing digestive problems. Consuming enough insoluble fiber promotes regularity of bowel movements and helps regulate blood sugar levels.

RESISTANT STARCH

Carbohydrates made up of high proportions of beta-glucose monomers (see right), such as cellulose, are referred to as resistant starches because they cannot be broken down by the small intestine. They pass into the large intestine, where they are fermented by gut bacteria.

This fermentation process produces short-chain fatty acids (SCFAs), which stimulate the immune system and can impact mental health.

Cooked and cooled potatoes and rice contain resistant starch, which is also found in whole grains like barley, oats, and sorghum, green bananas, and beans and legumes.

INCLUDING ENOUGH FIBER

Our average daily fiber intake is 10–15g, and we should aim for 28g. A food high in fiber is considered to have 5g fiber per serving.

Aim to include a mix of different sources of fiber. To ensure you get enough, include lots of whole grains, vegetables, fruits, beans, lentils, nuts, and seeds in your diet. aim for as wide a variety as possible.

Foods may contain a mixture of types of fiber. For instance, whole grain products are good sources of both insoluble fiber and resistant starch. Consuming a diet that includes fiber from whole grains may reduce your risk of developing heart disease, diabetes, and several types of cancers.

Bear in mind that suddenly increasing fiber can cause problems, such as bloating and loose bowel movements. Increase levels of fiber gradually and, if necessary, under the supervision of a doctor, dietitian, or nutritionist.

Cooked and cooled

COOLED COOKED WHITE RICE, POTATOES, SWEET POTATOES, OR PASTA PROVIDE MORE RESISTANT STARCH THAN IF CONSUMED HOT. Even if you reheat them later, the resistant starch content (see left) remains increased. So enjoy potato, pasta, and rice salads, and cook up extra batches to refrigerate and reheat for tomorrow's lunch or dinner. Care should be taken when storing cooked rice, which can contain bacterial spores that cause food poisoning. These spores flourish when rice is left to stand at room temperature, so cool and refrigerate rice within an hour of cooking, refrigerate for no longer than a day, and reheat until piping hot before consuming.

Starch and fiber

These are often confused, and easily so, since both are contained together in the same foods, and both are carbohydrates, made up of polysaccharides. But in starch, chains of glucose monomers (monosaccharides, see p.12) are joined by alpha bonds, which can be broken down in the small intestine. In fiber, glucose monomers are joined by beta bonds, which can't be broken down. Instead the chains remain intact throughout their passage through the small intestine.

weak alpha-bonds

strong beta-bonds

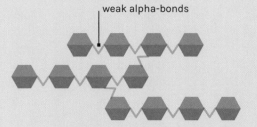

ALPHA-GLUCOSE MONOMERS

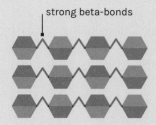

BETA-GLUCOSE MONOMERS

STARCH

Polysaccharides like amylopectin (found in rice, potato, white bread and pasta, wheat, and barley) are made with alpha-glucose monomers. The bond angles formed when alpha-glucose momomers join builds a branched and/or spiral structure. These bonds can be broken down by enzymes in the digestive system

FIBER

Polysaccharides like cellulose (found in plants) are made with beta-glucose monomers. The bond angles that form when these units of glucose join build into stable parallel chains that are strongly interlinked. There are no enzymes in the small intestine that are able to break down these beta-bonds.

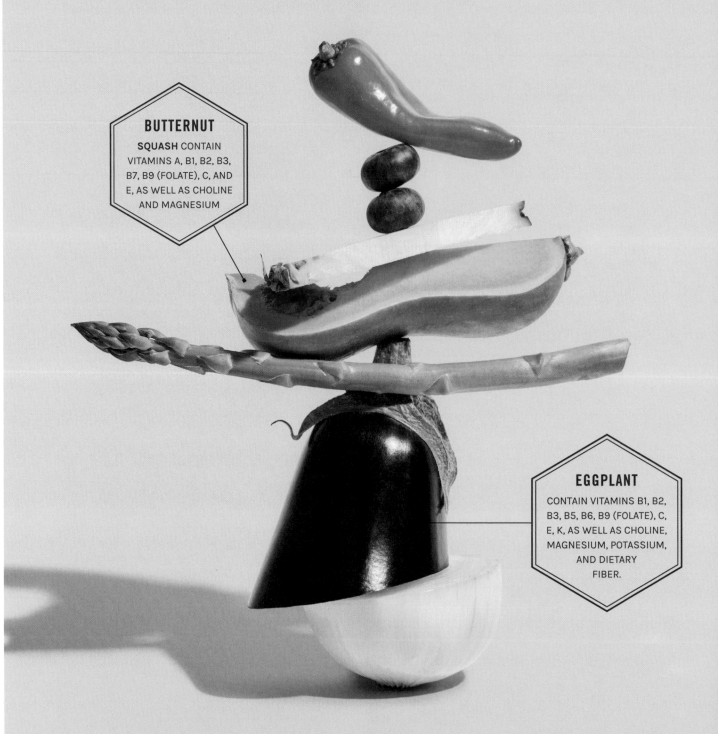

BUTTERNUT

SQUASH CONTAIN VITAMINS A, B1, B2, B3, B7, B9 (FOLATE), C, AND E, AS WELL AS CHOLINE AND MAGNESIUM

EGGPLANT

CONTAIN VITAMINS B1, B2, B3, B5, B6, B9 (FOLATE), C, E, K, AS WELL AS CHOLINE, MAGNESIUM, POTASSIUM, AND DIETARY FIBER.

WHAT ARE VITAMINS?

Vitamins are nutrients we need to obtain from the foods we eat in order to ensure optimal health and prevent nutritional deficiencies. Aim to include a colorful variety of veggies and fruits in your diet to pack in all the vitamins you need.

Our bodies cannot make all the micronutrients (see page 10) we need to function, so this requirement is met solely by diet. Most people enjoying a healthy, balanced diet will easily obtain enough vitamins. If you don't eat animal products, though, there are measures you can take to prevent potential nutritional deficiencies (see pp.130–131).

Vitamins come in two main forms, water-soluble and fat-soluble.

WATER SOLUBLE

Water-soluble vitamins are easily lost through bodily fluids (and in cooking) and must be replaced each day.

- **B vitamins** play an important role in keeping the nervous system healthy and helping our bodies release energy from the foods we eat. Folate (vitamin B9) helps with brain and spinal cord development in unborn babies (see page 178). **Sources** of B vitamins are:
  - **B1** Peas, bananas, nuts, whole grains
  - **B2** Milk, eggs, fortified cereals, mushrooms
  - **B3** Meat, fish, wheat flour, eggs
  - **B5** Chicken, beef, eggs, avocado
  - **B6** Pork, soybeans, peanuts, oats, bananas, milk
  - **B7** is needed in trace quantities, and is available from many food sources, so will be present in a varied and balanced diet
  - **B9** Leafy greens, chickpeas, edamame beans, broccoli, liver, foods fortified with folate
  - **B12** is found only in animal products, such as eggs, meat, or fish, or in fortified plant foods, such as some nutritional yeast products. If you are vegan, I highly advise reviewing whether you are getting enough B12.

- **Vitamin C** is often hailed as the cure to colds and flu because it contributes to healing. It also maintains healthy skin, blood vessels, and cartilage, and plays a role in the production of collagen, which maintains our skin's elasticity and strength. **Sources** include oranges, peppers, broccoli, bananas.

FAT SOLUBLE

Fat-soluble vitamins tend to accumulate within the body so are not needed in the diet on a daily basis.

- **Vitamins A and E** are powerful antioxidants, helping to protect cells from free radicals and aging. Vitamin A contributes to cell renewal and repair, but note that excesses during pregnancy may harm the baby (see page 183). Vitamin E reduces the effects of skin aging and the risk of skin cancer. **Sources** of vitamin A include carrots and sweet potatoes. **Sources** of vitamin E include almonds and avocados.

- **Vitamin D** is unique because it is a hormone that we can produce in our own bodies with exposure to sunlight. This means we don't need to get it from diet if there is enough exposure. However, with the use of sunscreen and the lack of sunlight in parts of the US and during winter, we are advised to supplement with vitamin D if our blood levels are low (see pages 138–139). **Dietary sources** include egg yolks, oily fish, fortified foods.

- **Vitamin K** is important for wound healing (we need it for blood clotting), and some evidence links it to bone health. **Sources** include green leafy vegetables, some cereal grains, and vegetable oil.

WHAT ARE MINERALS?

Our bodies need certain minerals to function well. Many foods contain
both vitamins and minerals, so a varied diet will help you meet
your mineral requirements.

Unlike vitamins, which are organic compounds (made by plants or animals), minerals are inorganic chemical elements that come from soil, rock, or water. They are absorbed from the environment by plants as they grow, and by animals that eat those plants. There are many minerals, each with benefits. Try to include each type in your diet regularly. You need some minerals in greater quantities, such as calcium, chloride, magnesium, phosphorous, potassium, sodium. Others, like iodine, iron,

selenium, and zinc are needed in trace quantities.

● **Calcium** is a vital component of bone and teeth, and a key nutrient for the nervous system, muscles, and heart. **Sources** include milk, yogurt, spinach.

● **Iodine** deficiency affects nearly one-third of the world's population. This mineral is essential for normal thyroid function and the production of thyroid hormones, which are involved in many processes in the body such as growth, brain

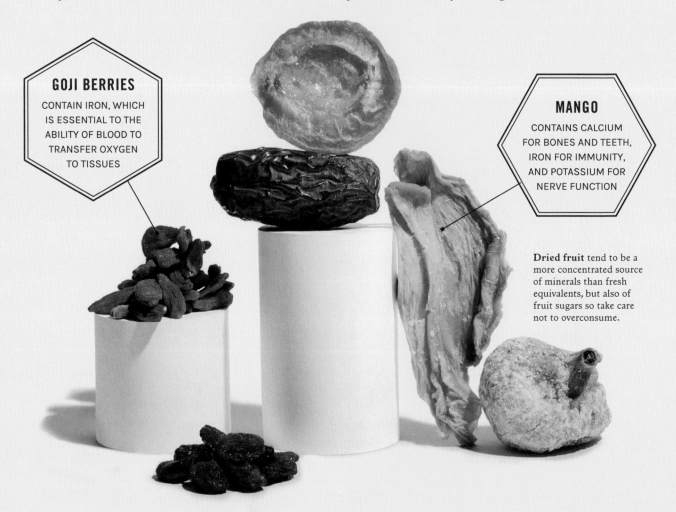

GOJI BERRIES

CONTAIN IRON, WHICH
IS ESSENTIAL TO THE
ABILITY OF BLOOD TO
TRANSFER OXYGEN
TO TISSUES

MANGO

CONTAINS CALCIUM
FOR BONES AND TEETH,
IRON FOR IMMUNITY,
AND POTASSIUM FOR
NERVE FUNCTION

Dried fruit tend to be a more concentrated source of minerals than fresh equivalents, but also of fruit sugars so take care not to overconsume.

development, and bone maintenance. Thyroid hormones also regulate the metabolic rate. **Sources** include fish, dairy products, eggs, seaweed.

● **Iron** deficiency is the most common nutritional deficiency in the world and the only one that is prevalent in developed countries. More than 30 percent of the world's population has anemia. Lack of iron lowers the ability of the blood to carry oxygen. Iron has many benefits, including improved immune and brain function. **Sources** include shellfish, broccoli, red meat, tofu.

● **Magnesium** plays a role in more than 600 cellular processes, including energy production, nervous system function, and muscle contraction. **Sources** include avocados, nuts, leafy greens.

● **Manganese** helps make and activate some of the enzymes in the body that carry out chemical reactions such as breaking down food. **Sources** include bread, nuts, breakfast cereals, green vegetables.

● **Potassium** is important for blood pressure control, fluid balance, and muscles and nerve function. **Sources** include bananas, spinach, potatoes, apricots.

● **Phosphorus** helps the body build strong bones and also release energy from food. **Sources** include red meat, dairy, fish, poultry, oats, bread.

● **Selenium** helps the immune system work correctly, prevents damage to cells and tissues, and promotes the health of the reproductive system. **Sources** include Brazil nuts, eggs, meat, fish.

● **Zinc** supports the immune system, hormone production, and fertility. It can help reduce skin inflammation and support wound healing and protects against UV damage from the sun. **Sources** include shellfish, red meat, eggs, chickpeas.

SHOULD I TAKE SUPPLEMENTS?

Food is the preferable way for the body to source nutrients, which are often better absorbed from foods than pills. It's possible for supplements to interact in ways that affect one another, or to contain one or more of the same nutrients, potentially leading to toxic buildups. Generally, water-soluble vitamins are less likely to cause harm than fat-soluble since they are excreted easily in your urine and have less chance of building up in the body. Yet be cautious. Too much vitamin C or zinc (a water-soluble mineral) may cause nausea, diarrhea, and stomach cramps. Too much selenium could lead to hair loss, gastrointestinal upset, fatigue, and mild nerve damage.

As the consequences of taking supplements can be serious, and supplements can be costly, it's not worth taking supplements unless advised to do so by a health care professional.

There are sometimes valid reasons for taking supplements, for instance, during preconception and pregnancy (see pages 178–181). Also, iron or vitamin B12 deficiency can lead to anemia. If you believe you have a nutritional deficiency, speak to your doctor. Blood tests can help diagnose deficiencies, and supplements can then be prescribed to help correct them.

IS HYDRATION PART OF NUTRITION?

Hydration is an incredibly important part of nutrition. Water is essential for all of the body's processes to work. In fact, we would survive a good deal longer without food than without water.

It is not easy to find even one system of the body that does not require water. Water enables the circulatory system to carry essential oxygen and nutrients to cells. Our kidneys need water to filter out waste products (see right). It helps us cool off via sweat when we are too hot. It helps the digestive system do its job. And the list goes on!

When it comes to the brain, 75 percent of its mass is water, so alongside the bodily processes, hydration also plays a crucial role in regulating mood, productivity, and concentration.

Your body uses a lot of water each day. You need to drink enough water to replace what is lost so the body continues to function well and you feel your best. So, drink up!

DAILY TARGETS

According to guidelines, most of us should aim to drink 2.7–3.7 liters of water every day. A typical mug or glass has a capacity of 7oz (200ml), so you'd need to have 11.5–15.5 drinks a day. Bear in mind that these are the recommended daily intake amounts and some people may need more. Aim for 15.5 cups (3.7 liters) daily if you easily get to 11.5 cups (2.7 liters). Get yourself a BPA-free reusable water bottle to help you keep track of your water intake.

Children and infants require less fluids than adults. Introduce tap water from the age of 6 months. With children, aim for 7–10 glasses a day.

Each kidney filters more than 100ml of blood per minute. Waste and excess water are separated from useful substances.

Blood in

Blood out

Each kidney contains roughly 1 million tiny filtering units called nephrons

Urine is directed along the ureter, a fine, muscular tube, to the bladder for storage until urination

Nephrons return useful substances to the blood supply

Nephrons create urine, a mix of waste substances and excess water

Ureter

Make adjustments to these targets based on your lifestyle. If you sweat a lot (say, if you're very active) you need to replenish that lost water frequently. On vacation in a hot climate, you may sweat more than usual and need to increase your water intake. Also, if you're breastfeeding, you require a lot of additional fluid. As we age, hydration is still important. Elderly people often struggle to get enough hydration due to issues

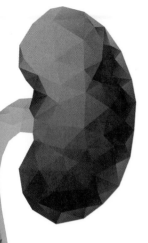

KIDNEYS

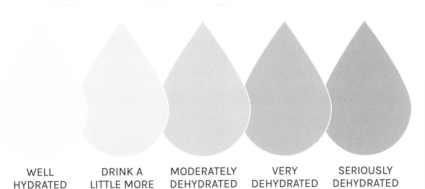

| WELL HYDRATED | DRINK A LITTLE MORE | MODERATELY DEHYDRATED | VERY DEHYDRATED | SERIOUSLY DEHYDRATED |

Urine color check
Urine should be quite clear in color. The darker yellow it is, the more dehydrated you are, and the more you need to drink to hydrate yourself.

with mobility and memory loss, for instance. It's important to note that people with these issues can feel more comfortable day to day by drinking plenty of water.

WHAT TO DRINK

About 20 percent of our total fluid intake comes from the food we eat. When it comes to the rest, research suggests that many people prefer to take in fluids in the form of sugary drinks, tea, coffee, and juices. In one survey, 23 percent of responders claimed they chose carbonated beverages to stay hydrated. Although these drinks supply you with necessary fluids, you also end up adding caffeine, sugar, and sweeteners (and their negative health effects)

to your body. The best way to hydrate is simply with water. In the US, tap water is safe to drink.

SIGNS OF DEHYDRATION

Signs of dehydration include dry mouth, dark yellow urine (see above), feeling tired, thirsty, and dizzy, and urinating fewer than four times per day. Studies show that at about 1 percent dehydration (equivalent to 1 percent of body weight water loss) there are negative effects on mental and physical function, which become more severe as dehydration increases.

Regularly underhydrating often leads to constipation. If you find that you are constipated frequently, try increasing your fluid consumption (see page 155).

Calculate your water needs

Use this calculation as a rule-of-thumb guide to help you calculate your daily water requirement. Make adjustments to factor in your sweat levels (based on the amount of physical activity you undertake).

 × 0.033 **=** Liters

YOUR WEIGHT (KG)

PER DAY

Example: you weigh 60kg, 60 x 0.003 = **1.98 liters**

BLADDER

WHAT IS DIGESTION?

Digestion is the process by which our bodies absorb the nutrients needed to stay alive from the foods we consume. Nutrients are passed into the bloodstream to be taken to wherever in the body they are needed, and waste matter is formed and excreted.

The digestive system is around 30ft (9m) long in adults, and an awful lot is achieved along this length. Each section of it plays an important role.

MOUTH

Food enters the mouth and is initially broken down by teeth as we chew it into smaller pieces. Digestive enzymes in saliva begin the process of chemically breaking down the food. The bolus (ball of masticated food) is swallowed and enters the esophagus.

ESOPHAGUS

At the back of the throat, behind the tongue, is the epiglottis, a flap of cartilage that covers the larynx (windpipe) as swallowed food passes it to enter the esophagus (food pipe). The esophagus is large muscular tube that extends from the epiglottis to the stomach. Its muscles move the bolus down the pipe to the stomach. The lower esophageal sphincter is a muscular ring acting as the stomach's gateway. Acid reflux results if it doesn't close properly.

STOMACH

The stomach releases digestive enzymes and acid that break down the food that enters. Gut muscles contract to churn the food, to help the chemicals break it up, and the acid kills off unwanted microbes in it. This process also informs the satiety hormone, leptin, to be released (p.105). (The corresponding hunger hormone, ghrelin, is released by the stomach when it is empty, to stimulate hunger pangs.) The stomach turns the food into chyme, which has a souplike consistency that the small intestine is able to process.

SMALL INTESTINE

The majority of nutrient absorption takes place in this 23ft (7m) long section of the digestive tract. It is covered with multiple tiny villi and microvilli that absorb nutrients from chyme through a process called diffusion (see pages 28–29) and pass them into the bloodstream.

Food spends 2–6 hours in the small intestine, being broken down by digestive enzymes so diffusion can take place. Some of these enzymes are supplied by the pancreas, which also releases hormones to help regulate blood sugar levels as they rise in response to eating a meal (pp.30–31). The gallbladder also secretes bile into the small intestine to further aid in digestion.

The remaining material consists mostly of water, bacteria, dead cells from the gut lining, and indigestible fiber (see page 18). It moves along the small intestine to the ileocecal valve —the gateway to the large intestine.

LARGE INTESTINE

The large intestine plays a key role in finishing the job and creating feces. During the 12–30 hours it spends in here, the initially liquid mixture that arrives is turned into stools as its water content is slowly absorbed by the large intestine.

The majority of the trillions of microbes living in the gut are in the large intestine. These gut bacteria seem to play an important role in the synthesis of key nutrients. They also communicate with our immune cells and help prevent inflammation. They ferment the indigestible fiber in the large intestine,

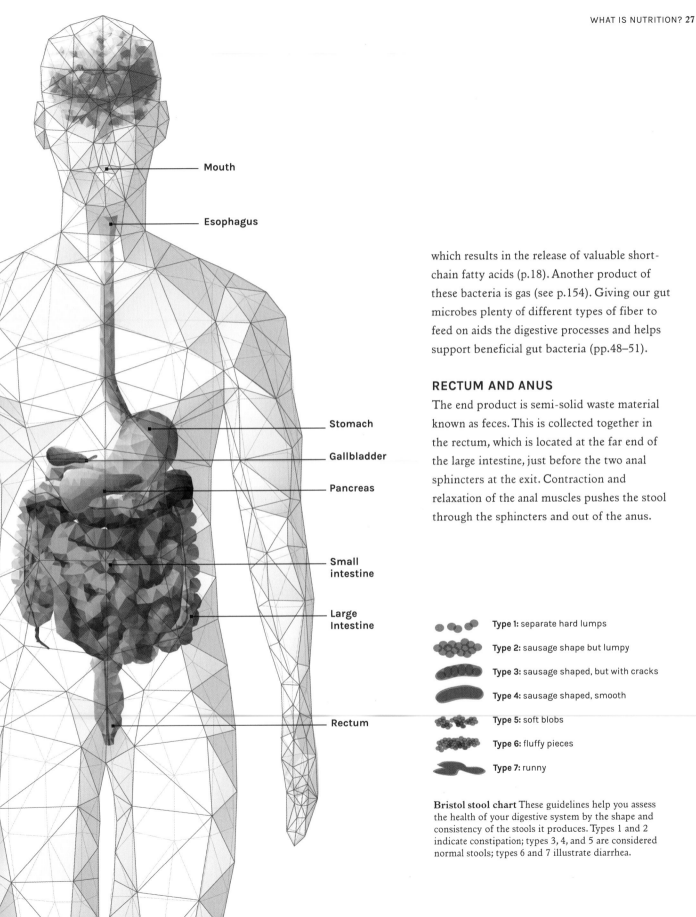

Mouth

Esophagus

Stomach

Gallbladder

Pancreas

Small intestine

Large Intestine

Rectum

which results in the release of valuable short-chain fatty acids (p.18). Another product of these bacteria is gas (see p.154). Giving our gut microbes plenty of different types of fiber to feed on aids the digestive processes and helps support beneficial gut bacteria (pp.48–51).

RECTUM AND ANUS

The end product is semi-solid waste material known as feces. This is collected together in the rectum, which is located at the far end of the large intestine, just before the two anal sphincters at the exit. Contraction and relaxation of the anal muscles pushes the stool through the sphincters and out of the anus.

Type 1: separate hard lumps

Type 2: sausage shape but lumpy

Type 3: sausage shaped, but with cracks

Type 4: sausage shaped, smooth

Type 5: soft blobs

Type 6: fluffy pieces

Type 7: runny

Bristol stool chart These guidelines help you assess the health of your digestive system by the shape and consistency of the stools it produces. Types 1 and 2 indicate constipation; types 3, 4, and 5 are considered normal stools; types 6 and 7 illustrate diarrhea.

HOW DOES THE BODY ABSORB NUTRIENTS DURING DIGESTION?

Once nutrients have been unlocked from the foods we eat by digestion (see page 26), they must be transferred into the bloodstream in order for the body to be able to use them. This process takes place in the stomach and the large and small intestines.

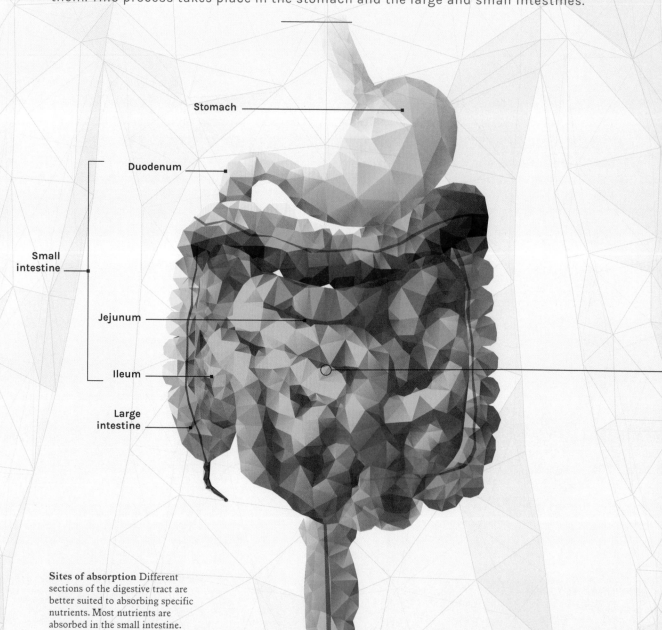

Stomach

Duodenum

Small intestine

Jejunum

Ileum

Large intestine

Sites of absorption Different sections of the digestive tract are better suited to absorbing specific nutrients. Most nutrients are absorbed in the small intestine.

The process by which nutrients are absorbed by the body is known as diffusion. The inner wall of the small intestine contains multiple tiny projections, called villi. These dramatically increase the surface area available for absorption to take place; the average small intestine has 2,690 sq ft (250 sq m) of surface area!

Villi are themselves covered in microscopic projections, known as microvilli, and these are responsible for diffusion. Nutrient particles released in the small intestine pass through these fine projections into the villi.

Each villi contains a mini-network of lymphatic vessels (lacteals) and capillaries that essentially connect the intestine to the body's circulatory and lymphatic systems. Proteins (broken down into amino acids) and carbohydrates (broken down into glucose) pass into the blood vessels. Fats (broken down into lipids) pass into the lymphatic vessels.

These blood and lymphatic vessels then transport those nutrients to different parts of the body to be used as needed or stored for later use.

STOMACH
water
ethyl alcohol
copper
fluoride
iodide
molybdenum

DUODENUM
calcium
biotin
copper
folate
iron
magnesium
niacin
phosphorous
riboflavin
selenium
thiamine
vitamins A, D, E, K

JEJUNUM
lipids
monosaccharides
amino acids
small peptides
biotin
calcium
chromium
folate
iron
phosphorous
magnesium
manganese
molydenum
niacin
pantothenate
riboflavin
thiamine
vitamins A, B6, C, D, E, K
zinc

ILEUM
bile salts
acids
folate
magnesium
vitamins B12, C
vitamins D, K

LARGE INTESTINE
water
short-chain fatty acids
biotin
potassium
sodium
chloride
vitamin K

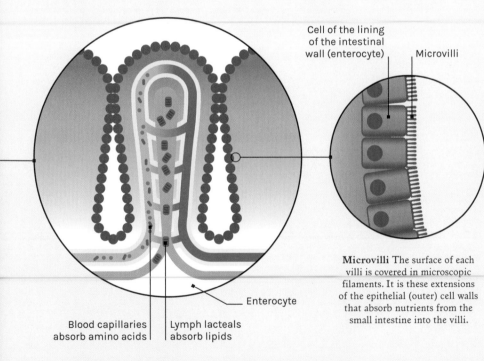

Cell of the lining of the intestinal wall (enterocyte)

Microvilli

Microvilli The surface of each villi is covered in microscopic filaments. It is these extensions of the epithelial (outer) cell walls that absorb nutrients from the small intestine into the villi.

Enterocyte

Blood capillaries absorb amino acids | Lymph lacteals absorb lipids

Villi These tiny fingerlike projections of the wall of the small intestine greatly expand its surface area. Each houses blood and lymphatic vessels that transport the nutrients absorbed by the villi to other parts of the body.

WHAT IS METABOLISM?

Metabolism is the term used to collectively refer to every single chemical reaction that takes place in your body in order to keep it alive. Metabolism is closely linked to nutrition, because the food we eat provides the energy required to fuel metabolism.

On average, we use 10 percent of energy intake on digestion itself, 20 percent on physical activity, and a whopping 70 percent by organs and tissues to keep the body alive. Every process in the body, from breathing to thinking, uses energy. A person's basal metabolic rate (BMR) is the number of calories needed to sustain their life while they are sitting still.

How the body metabolizes the energy it consumes is played out in a balancing act between two states—fed and fasted.

FED (ABSORPTIVE) STATE

During or after eating a meal, food is broken down and glucose (see pages 12–13) is released into the blood for cells to absorb and use as fuel. When the body has obtained more glucose from food than is needed by cells, they stop absorbing it. The resulting increase in blood glucose levels triggers the release of insulin. Insulin stimulates liver and muscle cells to reverse the conversion of glycogen into glucose (see pages 110–111) that takes place during the fasted state (see opposite) and, instead, absorb the surplus glucose in the bloodstream, convert it to glycogen granules, and store it for future use. Insulin also triggers the conversion of glucose to triglycerides (fats) in adipose tissue. Surplus fatty acids from the diet are also stored in adipose tissue.

How much energy gets stored in part depends on your BMR, which is influenced by factors such as genetics, age, sex, and body composition. To maintain a healthy and stable weight, we must (to simplify) put energy into the body that matches the energy expelled to stay alive, plus energy used in physical activity. If we consistently put in more calories than we burn, the excess is efficiently stored as fat.

FASTED (POSTABSORPTIVE) STATE

Several hours after eating, blood glucose levels drop, which triggers the pancreas to release glucagon (see opposite). This stimulates the liver and adipose tissue to metabolize glycogen stores, which releases glucose into the bloodstream to make it available for the body to use as energy.

After prolonged fasting, fat stores in adipose tissue are broken down into glycerol and fatty acids in the liver. Ketone bodies are a by-product of this reaction (see page 170). Protein is used for fuel only as a last resort (see page 33).

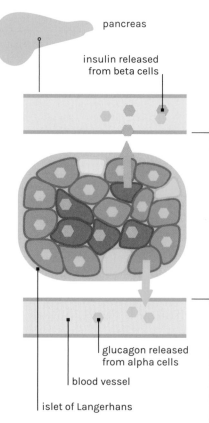

pancreas

insulin released from beta cells

Pancreatic cells

The pancreatic islets, also referred to as the islets of Langerhans, are clusters of cells that secrete the hormones responsible for balancing metabolism. These hormones work to balance blood sugar levels as the body oscillates between the fed and fasted states.

glucagon released from alpha cells

blood vessel

islet of Langerhans

What is a calorie?

Calorie is another word for kilocalorie (kcal), and 1 calorie is the amount of energy it takes to raise the temperature of 1g of water by 1.8°F (1°C).

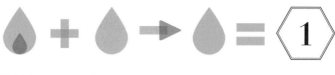

ENERGY   1G WATER 0°F   1G WATER 1.8°F   CALORIE (4.18KJ)

WHAT ARE CALORIES?

This unit of measurement is used to estimate how much energy there is stored in the chemical bonds of the foods we eat. Outdated guidelines state the average man needs about 2,500kcal a day to maintain a healthy weight, and for women, it's 2,000kcal. But these figures should be adjusted depending on factors such as age, size, and level of physical activity.

Your body may not gain the full amount of energy that is released from foods. Foods full of fiber, like nuts, for instance, take more energy to digest, and you absorb the remaining energy. Also, two people may absorb different levels of nutrients from the same quantity of the same foods. Gut health and the length of the intestines play a role in how much energy your body is able to absorb from foods.

It's important to remember that calories are not everything! A number definitely does not dictate how healthy you are or the quality of nutrition you consume. You could be in your body's ideal calorie-intake range by eating a chocolate brownie for breakfast, lunch, and dinner, but this won't provide you with all the key macronutrients, micronutrients, and fiber you need to be healthy and happy.

HIGH BLOOD SUGAR RESPONSE

| In response to high blood sugar levels, pancreatic beta cells release the hormone insulin into the bloodstream. | The presence of insulin enables glucose to enter the body's cells so that it can be used by them as energy. | As glucose in the bloodstream is depleted, blood sugar levels begin to fall, stimulating pancreatic alpha cells to release glucagon. |

BETA CELL   INSULIN   BLOOD SUGAR

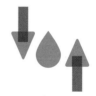

ALPHA CELL   GLUCAGON   BLOOD SUGAR

LOW BLOOD SUGAR RESPONSE

| In response to low blood-sugar levels, pancreatic alpha cells secrete the hormone glucagon. | Glucagon helps to regulate blood sugar by stimulating the release of glucose from stores in the liver and muscles. | The released glucose enters the bloodstream and is now available for use as energy. The resulting rise in blood sugar levels eventually stimulates pancreatic beta cells to release insulin. |

AM I MALNOURISHED?

Malnutrition is not something to worry about if you are receiving adequate nutrition from your diet. Sadly, this isn't the case for around 42 million people who are food insecure.

Social causes of malnutrition include poverty and lack of knowledge about nutrition. Physical causes include chronic or acute illness. For instance, an estimated 65–75 percent of people with Crohn's disease and up to 62 percent of those with ulcerative colitis are malnourished (see pages 164–165). Eating disorders may also be a cause (see page 210).

Malnutrition is most common in children and the elderly, and women are more impacted than men. As women have smaller musculature, they require 25 percent less energy per day than men but the same quantities of nutrients so must prioritize nutrient-rich foods, which is expensive. Pregnancy and breastfeeding also increase nutrient requirements.

Signs of malnutrition

BEING MALNOURISHED HAS A BIG IMPACT ON HEALTH AND LIFE QUALITY. SIGNS INCLUDE:

- increased incidence of illness and infection
- slower wound healing
- increased incidence of falls
- low mood
- reduced energy levels
- reduced muscle strength and muscle mass (see opposite)
- reduced quality of life
- reduced independence and ability to carry out daily activities
- deficiencies of multiple vital micronutrients (see pp.20-23).

If you have any concerns about malnutrition in you or a family member, see your doctor.

MALNUTRITION IN CHILDHOOD

Children with diseases and illness will often make up a large number of reported cases of childhood malnourishment. Food intolerances or allergies may prevent children from receiving adequate nutrition. Also, young children have small stomachs, so they need to eat more frequently than adults do in order to get in all the nutrients they need across the day. This can be difficult for parents to juggle, leading to malnourishment. Not growing or putting on weight as expected are key signs to look out for.

It's important to be mindful when discussing healthy weight with children. Even weighing children may be linked to future disordered relationships with food.

IDENTIFYING MALNUTRITION

Many people erroneously believe that only undereating causes malnutrition. In fact, the term refers to any severe imbalance of energy and nutrients in the body. This can describe a variety of malnutritional scenarios. Most obviously, the body may lack certain nutrients it needs to function in a healthy way. Toward the other end of the spectrum, energy intake (food) exceeds energy expenditure (physical activity). In the case of malnourishment due to obesity, the micronutrients needed for good health are often undersupplied due to a diet high in refined carbohydrates, snack foods, sugar, junk foods, and highly processed foods. Both undernutrition and overnutrition are forms of malnutrition, and both are detrimental to health.

According to the World Health Organization, 1.9 billion adults are overweight or obese, while 462 million are underweight.

Muscle wasting

If the amount of energy coming from the diet is inadequate for the body to perform basic functions, the body resorts to unlocking protein from muscles to use as energy. Over time, this reduces muscle mass, causing weakness and increasing the risk of injury.

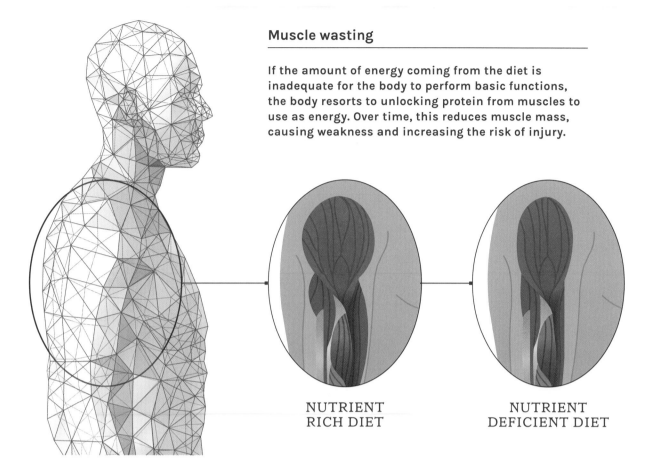

NUTRIENT
RICH DIET

NUTRIENT
DEFICIENT DIET

PHYSICAL IMPACT

When malnourished, vitamin and mineral deficiencies are more likely, which can impact negatively on many bodily processes. This could eventually affect a person's ability to undertake everyday tasks.

In the case of extreme undereating, once the body has depleted its glycogen stores (see page 110), it then turns to fat and protein stores for sources of energy. Reduced fat stores can lead to hormonal disruption. Women may lose their periods, and men can lose their morning erection. Once fat stores are depleted, breaking down protein to release amino acids to use as energy is the body's last resort. This leads to muscle wastage (see above). The mass of individual organs can also become depleted over time, affecting their function.

Malnutrition in childhood can stunt growth, lead to poor mental development, life-limiting behavioral abnormalities, and even life-threatening conditions.

Malnutrition in later life

UP TO ONE IN TWO ADULTS AGE 65 AND OLDER AND AS MANY AS 39 PERCENT OF OLDER ADULT PATIENTS MAY BE MALNOURISHED OR AT RISK.

In many cases, the overall energy intake is adequate, but there is too much fat, sugar, and salt in the diet and not enough fruit, vegetables, and oily fish, for instance. This may be due to entrenched habits, a reduced ability to cook, or increased pickiness; elderly people often lose their sense of smell and taste, which reduces appetite. Psychological factors, such as memory loss or dementia, can also contribute to reduced energy intake. A decline in gastrointestinal health means fewer nutrients are absorbed. Other physical issues, such as dysphagia (problems with swallowing) can limit energy intake.

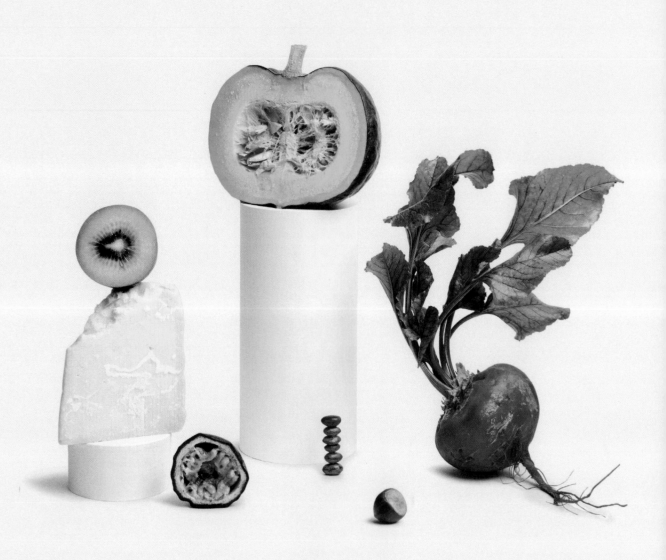

HOW CAN WE EAT WELL?

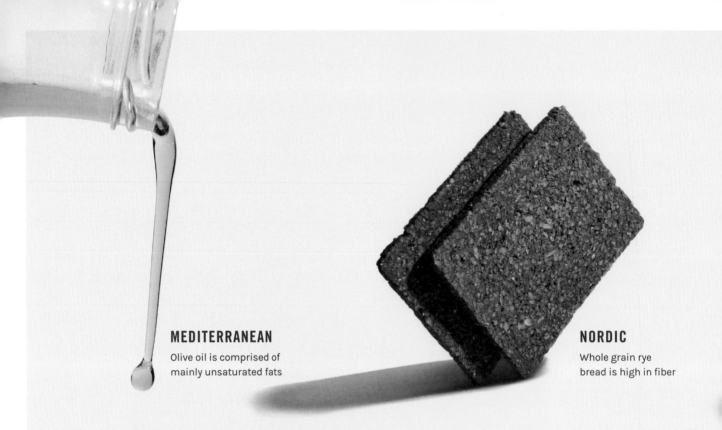

MEDITERRANEAN
Olive oil is comprised of mainly unsaturated fats

NORDIC
Whole grain rye bread is high in fiber

WHAT CAN I LEARN FROM MEDITERRANEAN, NORDIC, AND JAPANESE DIETS?

Noncommunicable diseases are now the leading cause of death globally, but in some parts of the world, people seem to live longer and healthier lives, which may be partly due to how they eat.

The **Mediterranean** diet concept developed when health organizations identified a possible link between traditional ways of eating in olive-growing areas like southern Italy and Greece and low levels of chronic disease among older people. The core focus is fresh, seasonal produce; plant-based eating; and healthy unsaturated fats, especially from olive oil. Vegetables, legumes (beans and lentils), whole grains, and nuts form the bulk of meals; moderate animal protein comes from oily fish and poultry; and there is low intake of red meat, eggs, yogurt, and cheese.

The **Nordic** diet was developed in response to rising obesity rates and to encourage people in the region to eat locally produced, sustainable foods. Most calories come from plant-based foods, making it fiber rich. Sea and lake fish and lean game meats are key protein sources, and canola oil, which is high in healthier monounsaturated fat, is used for cooking.

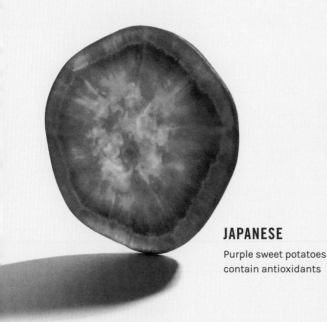

JAPANESE

Purple sweet potatoes
contain antioxidants

Sweet potatoes for life

OKINAWA, SOUTH OF MAINLAND JAPAN, HAS ONE OF THE WORLD'S LONGEST LIFE EXPECTANCIES, WITH A REPORTED 68 CENTENARIANS PER 100,000 INHABITANTS IN 2019.
While genetics, social habits, and exercise play a part, the islands' traditional diet relies heavily on purple sweet potatoes. These are high in fiber and a source of nutrients, including vitamins A and C and potassium, as well as the antioxidant anthocyanin, which various studies indicate helps protect against illnesses, including cardiovascular disease. Okinawans are also said to eat 18 different foods, including seven vegetables and fruits, every day.

Japan has among the highest life expectancy and lowest obesity rates globally. Its diet generally emphasizes plant-based eating of leafy vegetables, soybean-based foods like tofu and miso, and grains like rice and noodles, with animal protein from fish and pork. The Okinawa prefecture is particularly well known for longevity; its traditional diet is broadly similar, although high-fiber root vegetables are staples rather than rice, and very small amounts of fish and pork are eaten—not beef, eggs, or dairy.

ARE THESE DIETS HEALTHY?

Heart health: A variety of evidence suggests that the Mediterranean diet can reduce the risk of cardiovascular disease (CVD), meaning conditions affecting the heart or blood vessels. A landmark study found that the diet reduced both the number of heart attacks and strokes and all deaths from cardiovascular causes after five years. Research has linked Nordic eating to a reduction in major risk factors for CVD, including high blood pressure. Japan has lower rates of CVD than other developed countries; it may be that high consumption of soy-based foods and oily fish increases "good" HDL (high-density lipoprotein) cholesterol, which helps clear other types of cholesterol from the blood.

Cancer and diabetes: Studies suggest that closely following a Mediterranean diet long term may reduce the onset of various cancers (including breast, prostate, and colorectal). It's also been linked to improved control of blood glucose, which can help in managing type 2 diabetes. A strict Nordic diet has been associated with a lower risk of developing type 2 diabetes, although further research is needed.

Cognitive health: Japan has low rates of age-related diseases, although research hasn't yet identified the precise role of its diets. Most evidence focuses on Mediterranean eating, which has been linked to a slower rate of decline in memory and cognitive ability; high levels of plant antioxidants may reduce inflammation associated with diseases like Alzheimer's.

To find out how you could apply these diets to your daily eating, turn to pages 38–39.

HOW CAN I EAT A MORE MEDITERRANEAN, NORDIC, OR JAPANESE DIET?

Making small but sustainable changes that work with your personal preferences and budget is often the most effective way to eat a healthier diet. So how can you apply some of the key features of Mediterranean, Nordic, and Japanese eating?

DO I NEED TO EAT SWEET POTATOES?

Consuming purple sweet potatoes (or foods like seaweed or bitter melon, which are also featured in the Japanese diet) can provide positive nutritional benefits; however, it's better to eat them as part of a varied diet. Also, foods like these may need to be imported, increasing their cost and environmental footprint. You can find similar benefits to purple sweet potatoes in locally grown foods. For example, berries and cabbage are high in fiber, and red cabbage, blueberries, and blackberries are more accessible, and sustainable, sources of anthocyanins.

IS CANOLA OR OLIVE OIL HEALTHIER?

Olive oil has a superior reputation to canola oil because the Mediterranean diet is well researched. However, both contain monounsaturated fatty acids, known to be beneficial for heart health and cholesterol. Canola oil has less saturated fat and contains omegas 3, 6, and 9, which support brain, heart, and joint function, whereas olive oil, especially extra-virgin, is higher in antioxidant substances called polyphenols. Canola oil retains antioxidant properties and its neutral flavor at higher temperatures. Both oils are high in calories— around 120 calories per tablespoon for olive oil.

SHOULD I EAT MORE NUTS AND SEEDS?

Nuts and seeds are featured in both Mediterranean and Nordic eating; they are high in monounsaturated fat and protein and are sources of fiber and vitamins, making them a highly nutritious addition to a healthy and balanced diet. Their nutritional profile varies; for example, pecans are good for B vitamins and almonds for calcium, while Brazil, macadamia, and cashew nuts have a bit more saturated fat. Overall, they make a healthy snack or can be sprinkled on breakfast cereal or salad and vegetables. However, due to naturally high fat content, a palm-sized serving is one portion. Choose raw and unsalted varieties, if possible.

KEEP IT VARIED

While evidence points to some diets being more protective of health, it's not clear whether this is due to particular elements or the diet as a whole. This suggests there isn't one "perfect" diet; variety and a balance of healthy foods is probably more important.

What these diets share

Eating a wide range of different vegetables as the bulk of meals is the basis of all three diets, while other types of foods are common to at least two of them.

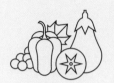   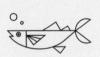

VEGETABLES AND FRUIT	WHOLE GRAINS	LEGUMES AND PULSES	LEAN AND OILY FISH	LEAN MEAT AND POULTRY	HEALTHY OIL

MEDITERRANEAN

EAT MOST
Vegetables; legumes and pulses (including chickpeas, kidney beans, fava beans, and lentils); whole grains (including whole wheat pasta); nuts and seeds

EAT MODERATELY
Fish (especially oily); poultry; olive oil; yogurt, cheese; fruit

EAT A LITTLE
Lean red meat; processed meat

KEY FEATURE
Olive oil (extra-virgin is highest quality)

TAKE NOTE
It is easy to follow, and the combination of foods have proven health benefits.

NORDIC

EAT MOST
Local vegetables, especially cabbage, peas, and root vegetables; local fruits and berries; whole grains (rye bread, oats, and barley); nuts and seeds

EAT MODERATELY
Sea/lake fish, including oily fish (herring, mackerel, salmon); low-fat dairy foods; canola oil

EAT A LITTLE
Lean red meat/game; poultry; eggs; cheese

KEY FEATURE
Canola oil (cold pressed is highest quality)

TAKE NOTE
Some root veggies, like potatoes, turnips, and parsnips, contain a lot of starchy carbs (pp. 12–13).

JAPANESE (OKINAWA)

EAT MOST
Local vegetables (including purple and orange sweet potato, Chinese okra, bitter melon, cabbage, seaweed, bamboo shoots)

EAT MODERATELY
Rice; noodles Soybean foods (including tofu and miso)

EAT A LITTLE
Fish and seafood; pork

KEY FEATURE
Purple sweet potatoes

TAKE NOTE
The diet is high fiber and low protein; the traditional version restricts some nutritious foods, like fruits and eggs.

WHAT ARE THE PRINCIPLES OF HEALTHY EATING?

There is so much information available and so many theories about the best way to eat well, you can easily end up feeling confused and frustrated. But the principles are simple—variety and balance on the plate.

There is no one way to achieve a healthy, balanced diet; it has to reflect your body's energy needs and your lifestyle, beliefs, and preferences. The "balanced plate" concept is a useful guide to the types and proportions of foods you should try to consume at mealtimes; apply it when shopping, cooking, or eating out to help you eat a varied, nutritious range of food.

It isn't essential to achieve the balance of food groups outlined here at every meal; just aim for it over the course of your day or week. A healthy adult's diet should contain carbohydrates, protein, and fat—in five key food groups. Hydration is also important; it helps you absorb nutrients and feel full.

WHAT'S ON A BALANCED PLATE?
● **Starchy carbohydrates** like rice, pasta, potatoes, quinoa, and oats should form the base of the meal and about one-third of your daily intake. Choose higher-fiber whole grain versions of these foods wherever possible, with reduced or no salt or sugar.

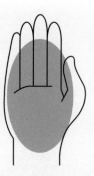

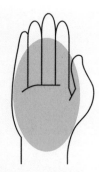

A good day's eating

Try to eat a range of foods from these groups daily and a small amount of high-fat, sugar, or salt foods only occasionally. Portion amounts shown here are based on an average woman, so they can vary; use your hands as a rough guide.

5+
PORTIONS OF FRUITS AND VEGETABLES

1 PORTION
= 1 handful/3oz/3-4 heaped teaspoons cooked spinach/green beans
= 1 medium tomato
= 1 medium apple/orange/banana
= 5oz of fruit juice (maximum per day)

3–4
PORTIONS OF STARCHY CARBOHYDRATES

1 PORTION
= 2 handfuls dried rice/pasta/couscous (less for 4 portions)
= 1 fist-size baked potato
= 2 slices bread

● **Vegetables and fruits** are just as important, if not more so; aim to eat at least five portions every day and exceed this wherever possible. Try to eat as wide a range as you can—this can include fresh, frozen, dried, and canned (in water or juice without salt or sugar). Include a higher ratio of vegetables to fruits and regularly change your combinations.

● **Protein-rich** foods include pulses (such as kidney beans, lentils, and chickpeas), quinoa, soybean products like tofu and tempeh, nuts, eggs, fish, and meat. It's best to limit the amount of red and processed meat (see pages 68–69).

● **Dairy** is a good source of many nutrients, including calcium and phosphorus; it includes hard and soft cheese, yogurt, and cow's milk.

6–8
GLASSES OF FLUIDS/DAY

Ideally water or sugar-free drinks; tea and coffee count

● **Unsaturated oils and fats** like olive oil or canola oil should be used in small amounts for cooking or to enhance flavor.

VEGETARIANS AND VEGANS

The same broad principles apply, but eating a wide variety of protein sources is even more important because most plant-based protein is incomplete, meaning it lacks certain essential amino acids (see pages 128–129).

Choose dairy alternatives like soy milk that are unsweetened and fortified with calcium, plus other sources of healthy omega-3 fatty acids like walnuts and ground flaxseed. Vegans may still need to supplement certain nutrients, such as vitamins D and B12, and iron (see pages 130–131).

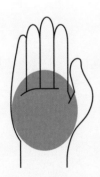

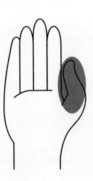

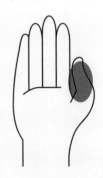

2–3
PORTIONS OF PROTEIN

1 PORTION
= half a handful salmon/chicken/steak
= 4oz cooked beans/lentils
= 1oz/palm-size nuts or seeds
= 3oz tofu

2–3
PORTIONS OF DAIRY AND ALTERNATIVE

1 PORTION
= 1oz/2 thumbs cheese
= 7oz low-fat cow's milk or unsweetened dairy alternative (4oz on cereal)
= 4oz low-fat yogurt

<1
SMALL AMOUNT OF FAT

= 1 teaspoon to cook a meal

SHOULD I EAT LESS MEAT AND MORE FISH?

Most adults choose meat over fish as their main source of protein, and most Americans eat less fish than recommended. But it's worth adding more into your diet because whether it's fresh, canned, or frozen, fish offers plenty of benefits.

A great source of protein, with less fat than many meats, fish and shellfish typically provide 15g–20g of protein per 100g, roughly a third of the daily recommended amount for many adults.

Eating fish—especially oily types like sardines, salmon, trout, and mackerel—is also a good way to obtain beneficial amounts of the omega-3 polyunsaturated fatty acids EPA (eicosapentaenoic acid) and DHA (docosahexaenoic acid). Oily fish is fattier than white fish and shellfish (some of which contain low levels of omega-3s), but it's mostly healthy polyunsaturated fat. EPA and DHA are associated with improved cardiovascular and cognitive health; for example, research indicates that oily fish eaters have more gray matter—the brain's major functional tissue linked to memory.

Many people don't eat enough omega-3s, which you can obtain only from diet. Some oily fish are also among the few dietary sources of Vitamin D (see pages 138–139).

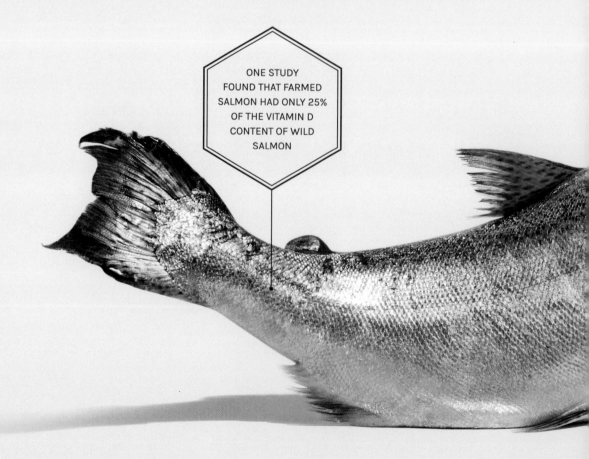

ONE STUDY FOUND THAT FARMED SALMON HAD ONLY 25% OF THE VITAMIN D CONTENT OF WILD SALMON

Dietary patterns that include regular fish consumption, like the Mediterranean diet, are generally associated with a lower risk of becoming overweight and obese. In a US-based study of more than 40,000 men, those who consumed more than one portion of any fish every week had a 15 percent lower risk of developing heart disease. The recommended portion for seafood is 8–10oz per week for adults 19 and older, 2–10oz for those 2–18 years old, and 2–3oz for children aged 6–23 months. US FDA and EPA guidelines suggest consuming seafood choices higher in EPA and DHA, such as salmon, anchovies, sardines, Pacific oysters, and trout, to limit mercury exposure.

BUYING AND COOKING

Unlike processed fish products, frozen and canned fish and seafood can be just as nutritious as fresh. Choose canned fish in water; brine contains a lot of salt, and omega-3s may seep into oil. Fish will absorb fats used during cooking, especially lean varieties. High-temperature methods can break down omega-3s—baking, grilling, and steaming will help preserve nutritional content. Sustainability is also a consideration (see pages 124–127).

WHAT ABOUT SUPPLEMENTS?

While it's not a substitute for fish within a balanced diet, fish oil can be beneficial for those who don't eat fish. However, it can contain heavy metals, and as fish derive omega-3 by eating algae, it may be better to opt for algae oil. Krill oil is extracted from crustaceans and is rich in both EPA and DHA. Fish liver oil contains a high amount of vitamin A; this may be harmful during pregnancy, and research suggests long-term use can weaken bones.

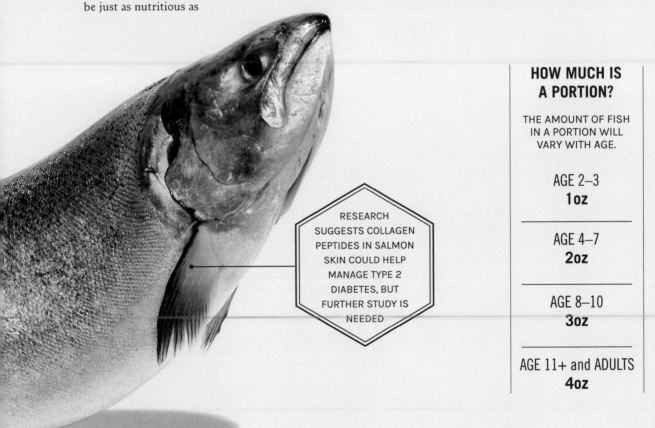

RESEARCH SUGGESTS COLLAGEN PEPTIDES IN SALMON SKIN COULD HELP MANAGE TYPE 2 DIABETES, BUT FURTHER STUDY IS NEEDED

HOW MUCH IS A PORTION?

THE AMOUNT OF FISH IN A PORTION WILL VARY WITH AGE.

AGE 2–3
1oz

AGE 4–7
2oz

AGE 8–10
3oz

AGE 11+ and ADULTS
4oz

WHY ARE LEGUMES AND PULSES SO GOOD FOR YOU?

Legumes and pulses provide variety of both flavor to the palate and nutrition to the body. They are packed full of micronutrients and fiber, and pulses specifically offer an affordable way to add nonmeat protein to your diet.

A legume is the leaves, stem, pod, or seeds of any plant from the Fabaceae family. We tend to eat the seed pods (like green beans and sugar snap peas) or the seeds from within them (either fresh, like peas and fava beans, or dried, like "pulses"). Both contain zero saturated fat and contain valuable nutrients.

There is strong evidence associating beans and lentils with a lower risk of cardiovascular disease, obesity, diabetes, and cancer. They are loaded with prebiotics (see pages 52–53) as well as fiber (see pages 18–19). Clinical trials show improved health outcomes in people eating 25–29g of fiber daily.

PULSES

The dried seeds of legumes are called pulses. They include lentils, chickpeas, black or pinto beans, soybeans, and kidney beans. These robust seeds contain varying amounts of the essential amino acids that make up protein (see pges 14–15). A 3.5oz (100g) serving of red lentils, chickpeas, or kidney beans provides 7.5g–8.5g of protein, which makes up a nice chunk of your daily requirement. You can save much money by getting more of your protein from beans rather than meat, adding lots of valuable fiber to your diet at the same time. Being starchy carbs (see pages 12–13), they typically contain around 8g fiber per 100g—that's almost one-third of your daily requirement.

LEGUMES

Eating leguminous vegetables like green beans is also important, because they contain other important nutrients. There is a lot of research to suggest we should aim to include more leguminous vegetables in our diet. Aim to include more green beans, butter beans, and soybeans in your diet.

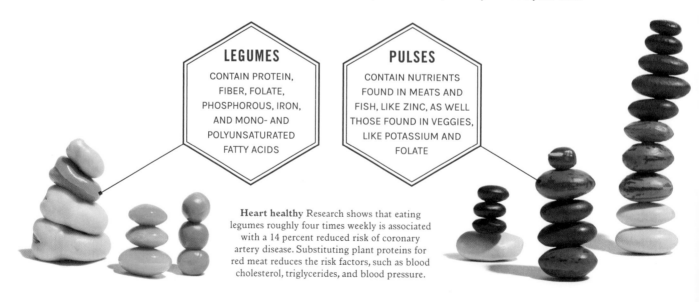

LEGUMES

CONTAIN PROTEIN, FIBER, FOLATE, PHOSPHOROUS, IRON, AND MONO- AND POLYUNSATURATED FATTY ACIDS

PULSES

CONTAIN NUTRIENTS FOUND IN MEATS AND FISH, LIKE ZINC, AS WELL THOSE FOUND IN VEGGIES, LIKE POTASSIUM AND FOLATE

Heart healthy Research shows that eating legumes roughly four times weekly is associated with a 14 percent reduced risk of coronary artery disease. Substituting plant proteins for red meat reduces the risk factors, such as blood cholesterol, triglycerides, and blood pressure.

WHY ARE WHOLE GRAINS SO GOOD FOR YOU?

Humans across the globe consume plenty of cereal crops, such as barley, oats, rice, and wheat. It is the seed of these crops, known as the grain, that we eat. Whole grains are those left intact when prepared for use as an ingredient.

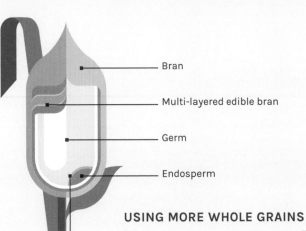

Bran

Multi-layered edible bran

Germ

Endosperm

WHOLE GRAINS
INCLUDE WILD AND BROWN RICE, WHOLE OATS AND RYE, QUINOA, CORN, FREEKEH, AMARANTH, SORGHUM, AND TEFF

When they are being processed, refined carbohydrates have the bran and germ removed, which results in light flours for making white bread or fluffy cakes, or enables the production of white rice and white pasta. However, the bran and germ are valuable sources of fiber and nutrients. While refined carbs provide energy (see page 12), whole grains are 75 percent more nutritious.

Whole grains provide fiber, B vitamins, omega-3 fatty acids, protein, as well as many antioxidants, micronutrients, and phytochemicals. Regular consumption is linked to gut and heart health and the prevention of cancers, diabetes, and obesity. Surveys show that 95 percent of adults don't eat enough whole grains, and almost one in three adults get none at all.

USING MORE WHOLE GRAINS

In many cases, you can swap out refined products for whole grain ones—substitute whole wheat bread for white bread, or brown rice for white rice. Try serving a curry with a new and whole grain, like buckwheat, spelt, or pot barley, for instance.

Whole oats, for example, are also very nutritious. Try having oatmeal for breakfast more frequently, and choose granola bars for snacks.

From time to time, experiment with new whole grains to consider how you might add more types to your culinary repertoire. Some are sweeter, like farro. Some make great accompaniments to a main dish, like quinoa or bulgur. There's tons of fantastic advice and inspiration on social media to help you get started with new flavors.

SHOULD I COOK MEALS FROM SCRATCH MORE OFTEN?

Cooking a meal using fresh, canned, or frozen ingredients can seem like a chore, especially when life is already busy. Is it worth the extra time and effort— and does it actually work out more expensive, as many people assume?

Preparing and cooking meals yourself can have real health benefits because you are in charge of how much sugar, fat, and salt goes into your meal (see pages 64, 66, and 70). Many highly processed foods, in particular ready-made meals and takeout, have added salt for flavor and preservation and are cooked in a significant amount of oil or butter, not to mention the addition of sugar to entice people into eating more of them (see pages 58–59). Cooking your own meals also means you can choose more nutrient-dense ingredients. For example, try using whole grains instead of refined carbohydrates, such as brown rice rather than white or whole wheat pasta or couscous (see pages 12–13).

How you cook matters

Potatoes are a rich source of micronutrients like potassium, vitamin B6, and vitamin C. How you prepare and cook them, like other ingredients, can significantly alter their nutritional content (shown per 3.5oz) and affect nutrient loss.

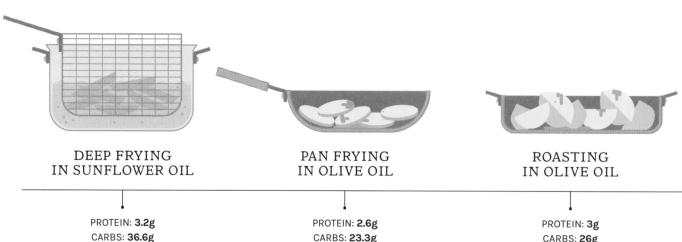

DEEP FRYING IN SUNFLOWER OIL

PROTEIN: **3.2g**
CARBS: **36.6g**
FAT: **14.5g**

During deep frying, fat penetrates the flesh; deep-fried potatoes can have 2–3 times the calories of boiled or baked.

PAN FRYING IN OLIVE OIL

PROTEIN: **2.6g**
CARBS: **23.3g**
FAT: **7g**

Quick frying has little impact on protein or mineral content, retains vitamin C, and boosts fiber by forming resistant starch.

ROASTING IN OLIVE OIL

PROTEIN: **3g**
CARBS: **26g**
FAT: **4.5g**

This flavorful method provides more calories than most others but is healthier than deep-fat frying.

HOME COOKING AND HEALTH

A body of research supports the benefits of cooking from scratch. One 2017 study found that people who ate home-cooked meals more than five times a week were 28 percent less likely to have an overweight BMI (body mass index) score compared with people eating this way less than three times weekly. They also ate more fruits and vegetables. Research also suggests that cooking improves self-esteem and mood, although there are many factors to consider when isolating studies. Creating meals addresses different aspects of psychological well-being by providing a sense of autonomy and confidence and opportunities to socialize and build relationships.

COST-EFFECTIVE COOKING

Cooking with fresh ingredients like meat and fish can still work out cheaper than buying preprepared and takeout meals. Keep these simple tips in mind:

● Use less meat and bulk up stews, soups, and curries with protein-rich canned beans, whole wheat pasta, and brown rice.

● Divide your usual portion of meat into two meals, for instance, by adding grated carrot, zucchini, or chopped mushrooms. Loose vegetables are often less expensive.

● Switch fresh fish for cheaper frozen or canned, ideally in plain water. Frozen fish has just as many, or even more, nutrients as fresh. This is true for many other ingredients.

● Shop with a friend to split bulk-buy discounts and bargains nearing sell-by dates. Separate large packs of meat or fish into portions and freeze ones you won't cook before the use-by date.

● Before shopping, plan your meals and check which ingredients are already in your pantry.

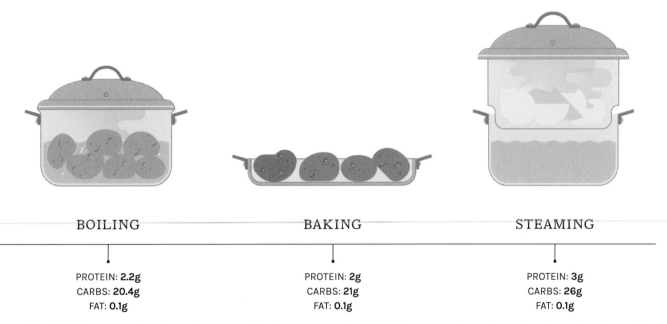

BOILING

PROTEIN: **2.2g**
CARBS: **20.4g**
FAT: **0.1g**

Boiling with skins on greatly reduces the loss of water-soluble micronutrients, like vitamins B6 and B12, into cooking water.

BAKING

PROTEIN: **2g**
CARBS: **21g**
FAT: **0.1g**

Baked potatoes are virtually fat-free, and baking in skin is one of the best methods for retaining nutrients.

STEAMING

PROTEIN: **3g**
CARBS: **26g**
FAT: **0.1g**

Steaming retains the most nutrients; it is particularly useful for new potatoes, which are high in water-soluble vitamin C.

WHAT IS GOOD GUT HEALTH, AND WHY IS IT IMPORTANT?

A healthy gut isn't just necessary for good digestion. Scientists are uncovering more about all the ways the bacteria in your gut may be involved in your overall health—even your mental well-being.

We tend to associate bacteria with infection, but most bacteria in the gut are actually beneficial. Along with yeasts, fungi, and viruses, bacteria make up the gut microbiome—the ecosystem of around 100 trillion microorganisms mainly found in the colon. There are around 1,000 species of gut bacteria; the specific combination is unique to each of us and changes over our life span. Research suggests maintaining a balance between more and less helpful bacteria is key to a healthy gut.

In addition to digesting food, gut bacteria perform many other important tasks. For example, they help absorb minerals from food, synthesize vitamins like vitamin K (which helps with blood clotting), and digest dietary fiber, releasing molecules, including butyrate, which contributes to a stronger gut barrier, and propionate, which helps the liver regulate blood sugar levels and appetite.

WIDER HEALTH

People with the inflammatory bowel conditions Crohn's disease and ulcerative colitis have been found to have fewer species and a lower proportion of beneficial gut bacteria. Studies have also observed lower diversity in people with obesity, diabetes, and certain types of eczema and arthritis. Dysbiosis—an imbalance in the gut microbiome—has also been shown to contribute to metabolic syndrome, allergies, colorectal cancer, and Alzheimer's disease. A healthy gut supports the immune system—

around 70 percent of immunity-related cells are located there. Friendly bacteria interact with the intestinal lining to prevent harmful molecules from leaking into the body and help activate new immune cells (see pages 136–137).

HEALTHY GUT, HEALTHY MIND?

We know the brain affects the gut because we often feel stress or excitement in our stomach, but diet could also have an impact on our brain. Scientists have only recently started exploring the mechanisms by which gut bacteria may influence the brain—and therefore how gut health could affect mood. Several studies have found the microbes of people with depression differ from others; in 2019, scientists identified two specific types of gut bacteria (*Coprococcus* and *Dialister*) that were consistently lacking in the microbiomes of the depressed subjects.

Fermenting discomfort

FERMENTATION IS WHEN THE GUT BACTERIA BREAK DOWN DIETARY FIBER.

This creates hydrogen and methane gas, which is normal and in fact shows that the gut is working effectively. However, those with a functional gut disorder like irritable bowel syndrome are more susceptible to the effects, due to increased sensitivity of their intestines—so they can feel bloating or abdominal pain.

Brain nuclei produce
serotonin to affect mood

The vagus nerve links
organs to the medulla

NEURO-TRANSMITTERS

CHEMICAL MESSAGES
LET THE BRAIN AND
BODY COMMUNICATE
AND PROMPT OR
INHIBIT FEELINGS

VAGUS NERVE

THIS NERVE DIRECTLY
CONNECTS THE BRAIN
TO THE GUT'S OWN
NERVE CELLS AND
SENDS SIGNALS
BOTH WAYS

IMMUNE SYSTEM

THE GUT IS THE MAIN
LOCATION FOR
EXPOSURE TO MANY
FOREIGN PATHOGENS
LIKE TOXINS AND
VIRUSES

Serotonin is a neurotransmitter
mostly made in the gut to
promote feelings of fullness and
control appetite; it may also
reach the brain via the blood and
influence levels of happiness.

As a main communication
highway between the brain and
numerous organs, its functions
include regulating heart rate,
digestion, fighting inflammation,
and relaxation.

Gut bacteria stimulate the
production of specific cells that
fight infection; it is thought that
these could travel via the blood or
lymph and interact with the
central nervous system.

Nerve cells in the gut
lining control digestion/
elimination

Gut mucous membranes
are an important site of
immune activity

The gut–brain axis

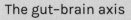

**Scientists now know there
is a constant two-way
communication between the
gut and brain that happens
via different pathways—
including the vagus nerve,
cells of the immune system,
and chemicals released into
the bloodstream.**

The vagus nerve's other
end point is in the colon

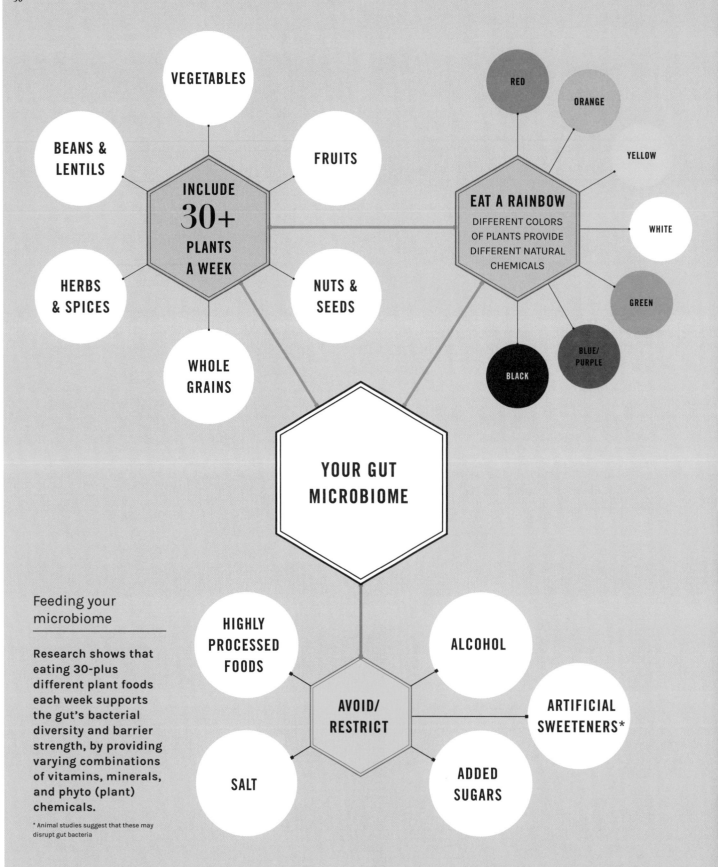

50

VEGETABLES

BEANS & LENTILS

FRUITS

INCLUDE 30+ PLANTS A WEEK

HERBS & SPICES

NUTS & SEEDS

WHOLE GRAINS

RED

ORANGE

YELLOW

EAT A RAINBOW
DIFFERENT COLORS OF PLANTS PROVIDE DIFFERENT NATURAL CHEMICALS

WHITE

GREEN

BLACK

BLUE/ PURPLE

YOUR GUT MICROBIOME

Feeding your microbiome

Research shows that eating 30-plus different plant foods each week supports the gut's bacterial diversity and barrier strength, by providing varying combinations of vitamins, minerals, and phyto (plant) chemicals.

* Animal studies suggest that these may disrupt gut bacteria

HIGHLY PROCESSED FOODS

ALCOHOL

AVOID/ RESTRICT

ARTIFICIAL SWEETENERS*

SALT

ADDED SUGARS

HOW CAN I INCREASE GUT MICROBIOME DIVERSITY?

The key to a healthy, functioning gut is the diversity of the bacteria living in it. Although our gut microbiome is established in infancy, as adults, we may still be able to boost our good gut bacteria through the foods we choose.

Our gut microbiome is shaped from birth to around three years old. Most microbes come from the mother's birth canal during vaginal birth, or from the hospital environment in a Cesarean section, and also vary with breast or bottle feeding. Infants then acquire bacteria from their environment, nearby people, and diet. Once established, our lifestyle, stress levels, and diet can still cause shifts in our microbiome that may support or undermine health. For example, some strains from the *Bifidobacteria* and *Lactobacillus* families can prevent potentially harmful gut bacteria from getting out of control.

DIVERSITY MATTERS

Bacterial diversity is associated with how many unique plant species we eat, according to an international gut microbiome project analyzing data from thousands of volunteers. Researchers identified that eating 30-plus types of plants a week is linked to the production of various short-chain fatty acids; these help protect both gut health and immunity.

Eating plenty of indigestible fiber has also been shown to boost the richness of the gut microbiome, while a low level in the diet reduces overall bacterial diversity. As well as many vegetables, whole grains like oats, brown rice, beans and lentils, and nuts and seeds are good fiber sources—US health guidelines advise healthy adults eat 28g of fiber on a 2,000-calorie diet. Many have a "prebiotic" effect by feeding beneficial bacteria. Naturally fermented "probiotic" foods like kefir can also be helpful; for example, most species of *Lactobacillus* are found in fermented foods (see pages 52–53).

In contrast, several studies have found that a typical Western diet, which is high in animal protein and fat and low in fiber, led to a marked decrease in total numbers of bacteria and beneficial *Bifidobacteria*. Some have also noted that while a change in diet can rapidly alter microbiome balance, it takes a long-term change in eating habits to create significant shifts in bacterial diversity.

MEDICATIONS

Overuse of medications, particularly antibiotics, can decrease the amount of good bacteria in the gut. In one study, more than a quarter of 900 antibiotic medications tested were found to be potentially damaging to the growth of gut microbes. Probiotics can help increase good bacteria in the gut; the most evidence we have for their effectiveness is taking them after a course of antibiotics to prevent antibiotic-associated diarrhea.

Fecal transplant

THIS PROCEDURE IS A FORM OF BACTERIOTHERAPY THAT USES A STOOL FROM A HEALTHY DONOR. It is placed in the colon of someone who is unwell in order to rebalance their gut bacteria. Although this is still a developing area, a 2016 review found its success rate varied from a third to three-quarters of cases in trials involving irritable bowel syndrome patients. While this is a developing area and research is ongoing, several studies indicate it may be an effective treatment for recurring *C. difficile* infections.

WHAT IS THE DIFFERENCE BETWEEN PRE- AND PROBIOTICS?

The concept of consuming a daily prebiotic or probiotic to keep your gut balanced and healthy is hugely popular—sales of probiotic supplements alone have been projected to hit $65 billion by 2024. But is it really that straightforward?

Probiotics are live strains of bacteria consumed to directly increase the population of "good" bacteria in the gut. Prebiotic foods feed existing gut bacteria so they can thrive and work effectively.

Probiotics are found in several fermented foods and drinks—specially formulated probiotic drinks, yogurts, and supplements contain specific "friendly" bacterial strains, often from the *Lactobacillus* and *Bifidobacteria* species.

One concern around probiotic foods is how many microbes can survive the acidic conditions in the stomach in order to reach your colon intact and colonize there. Live strains will also be destroyed by heat-based processes like canning or pasteurizing. There are no clear guidelines on how much you need to eat to gain a benefit from probiotics. In the US, the probiotic supplement market is largely unregulated. Bacteria content of supplements is specified on the label as "CFU" (colony forming units).

WHAT ARE THE BENEFITS?

Research suggests probiotics are mainly of benefit when your gut microbiome is out of balance, for instance, to relieve diarrhea caused by infection or after a course of antibiotics. Although studies are limited, certain types of bacterial strains have been found to reduce symptoms of irritable bowel syndrome, particularly bloating. Otherwise, a study found that eating fermented foods 1–5 times weekly is associated with a subtle change in gut bacteria. In general, though, healthy people should not require probiotic supplements.

A key benefit of prebiotic foods is that different types of the nondigestible fibers within the food are broken down by gut bacteria, which then produces gut protective short-chain fatty acids. Some studies show that eating a type of dietary fiber called inulin can help maintain the gut's mucus barrier and prevent inflammation. It's best to increase prebiotic food intake gradually, to avoid bloating.

Prebiotics

MANY NATURALLY PREBIOTIC FOODS AND DRINKS WILL ALSO PROVIDE VARIOUS VITAMINS, MINERALS, AND PHYTOCHEMICALS.

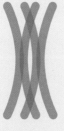

FIBER

FRUITS
APPLES
DATES
PRUNES
DRIED MANGO
PEARS
GRAPEFRUIT
APRICOT

VEGETABLES
LEEKS
GARLIC
LEGUMES/PULSES
(BEANS & LENTILS)
JERUSALEM ARTICHOKE
CHICORY ROOT
ASPARAGUS

OTHERS
WHEAT BRAN
CASHEWS
PISTACHIOS
CHAI TEA
FENNEL TEA

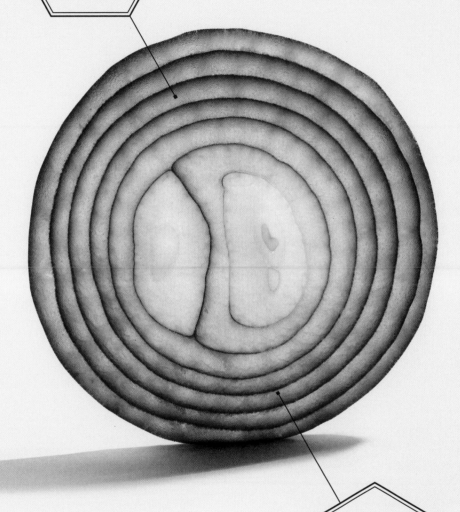

ONIONS CONTAIN DIFFERENT TYPES OF NONFERMENTABLE FIBERS THAT CONVERT TO BENEFICIAL SHORT-CHAIN FATTY ACIDS IN THE COLON

Raw benefits: To obtain more of a prebiotic benefit, onion and garlic can be eaten uncooked, if possible.

ALLIUMS

AS WELL AS PREBIOTIC PROPERTIES, ONIONS, LEEKS, AND GARLIC ARE A RICH SOURCE OF ANTIOXIDANTS

Probiotics

PROBIOTICS ARISE FROM LACTOFERMENTATION, WHERE CULTURES FEED ON STARCH OR SUGARS IN THE FOOD AND CREATE LACTIC ACID.

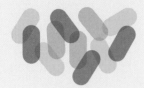

BACTERIA

YOGURT

YOGURT IS MADE FROM MILK FERMENTED BY BACTERIA; FOR PROBIOTIC EFFECT, CHOOSE ONE WITH LIVE OR ACTIVE CULTURES AND NO ADDED SUGAR.

KEFIR

THIS DRINK IS A POTENT PROBIOTIC THAT CAN BE MADE AT HOME FROM MILK OR WATER AND REUSABLE "GRAINS" COMBINING BACTERIA, YEAST, AND ENZYMES.

SAUERKRAUT

MADE FROM CABBAGE THAT HAS BEEN FERMENTED USING NATURALLY PRESENT LACTIC ACID BACTERIA, SAUERKRAUT IS ALSO A GOOD SOURCE OF FIBER.

KIMCHI

KIMCHI IS A WIDELY USED CONDIMENT IN KOREA THAT CONSISTS OF CABBAGE OR OTHER VEGETABLES FERMENTED BY BACTERIA, OFTEN FLAVORED WITH CHILE AND GARLIC

KOMBUCHA

MADE FROM SWEET TEA FERMENTED WITH A CULTURE OF BACTERIA AND YEAST, RESEARCH ON ITS BENEFITS ISN'T CLEAR.

WHAT ARE THE ELEMENTS OF A POOR DIET?

A poor diet is one that isn't providing enough crucial nutrients to keep you in optimal health, or your body's energy needs and your appetite in balance. Over the long term, it could also have life-limiting effects.

A key way of defining a poor diet is one that is high in salt, sugar, and saturated fat. US health guidelines recommend a daily intake of <2,300mg of sodium, <10% total calories of added sugar, and <10% total calories of saturated fat (pp. 64, 66, and 70). Preprepared food is responsible for much of the excess; three-quarters of the salt in our diet comes from processed foods, including staples like bread, while three large slices of takeout vegetable pizza could contain around 12g of salt. But fast food is only one factor—adding a tablespoon of soy sauce to a healthy vegetable stir-fry could increase its salt content by up to 3g.

Poor diet is not only about eating too much of the "wrong" foods; it can also mean not consuming enough nutrient-dense foods. In 2017, a global study of diet and mortality found that eating low amounts of healthy foods—including whole grains, fruits and vegetables, and nuts and seeds—was associated with more deaths than a diet with too much salt, sugar-sweetened drinks, red and processed meats, and trans fats. A low intake of whole grains was the single dietary factor associated with most deaths in the US and western Europe. Of course, multiple lifestyle factors can contribute to poor health, but diet is an area where people can take some control.

HEALTH IMPLICATIONS

The same study estimated that one in five deaths worldwide were associated with eating a poor diet, with cardiovascular disease (including heart disease, heart failure, and stroke) the leading global cause of diet-related deaths.

Poor diet is mainly associated with weight gain. In the US, three-quarters of adults are classed as overweight or obese, and more than half have at least one preventable chronic disease related to diet. While excess body fat is often not a choice, people with obesity are three times more likely to develop colon cancer and five times more likely to develop type 2 diabetes. The World Health Organization (WHO) wants to reduce the adult global population's intake of salt by 30 percent to halve cases of diabetes and stroke by 2025, due to the association between excess salt and raised blood pressure (see pages 70–71).

SHOULD I EAT FEWER CALORIES?

In terms of overall calories, recommended daily adult intakes in the US are 2,000 for women and 2,500 for men. Chronic overconsumption may lead to unhealthy body fat levels and increase the risk of developing type 2 diabetes, heart disease, and some cancers. However, occasionally eating more calories than you need is unlikely to impact your health. Instead of focusing simply on the number of calories, consider whether you have enough variety in your daily diet and its quality as a whole.

Healthier meal hacks

Don't automatically rule out meals you enjoy, but be aware they could be high in salt, sugar, and fat and low in fiber or protein. Some simple changes can improve a meal's potential nutritional value and keep you feeling satisfied.

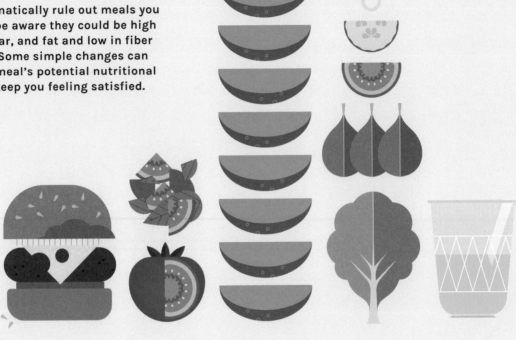

BUN (fiber)
- ✔ WHOLE WHEAT BUN, **3.4g**
- ✗ WHITE BUN, **1.1g**

BURGER (saturated fat)
- ✔ VEGETARIAN BEAN BURGER, **1.2g**
- ✗ BEEF BURGER, **11.6g**

FRIES (fat/serving)
- ✔ BAKED SWEET POTATOES, **3.7g**
- ✗ FRENCH FRIES, **6.6g**

SAUCES (sugar/serving)
- ✔ HOMEMADE SALSA, **0.1g**
- ✗ KETCHUP, **3.4g**

EXTRAS (micronutrients)
- ✔ SPINACH, ONION & TOMATO > PLAIN LETTUCE

DRINK (sugar/3.5oz)
- ✔ SPARKLING WATER WITH SPLASH OF JUICE, **4.7g**
- ✗ SUGAR-SWEETENED BEVERAGE, **10.6g**

EXPANDING PORTIONS

THE PORTION SIZE ON THE PACK OF AN AVERAGE MUFFIN ROSE FROM **85g** OVER A DECADE TO AS MUCH AS **130g**

WHY DO SO MANY OF US HAVE POOR DIETS?

The reasons people don't eat a healthy, balanced diet are complex and often interlinked. They can range from access to a wide choice of different foods to psychological influences they may not even be aware of.

Lack of education about food, and an unhealthy relationship with it, are key factors contributing to poor diets in developed countries. Giving sweets to an upset child arguably creates an emotional association; as an adult, that person is more likely to reach for sugary carbohydrates to self-soothe against stress or anxiety. Animal and human studies show that certain foods, especially those high in fat, carbohydrates, and salt, stimulate the brain's reward centers. The Yale Food Addiction Scale was developed to identify markers relating to certain foods, although this is a controversial area with conflicting research. But evidence clearly shows that the more highly palatable the food, the more likely it is to be consumed for pleasure—called "hedonic" eating (see pages 58–59). Manufacturers design the specific flavors and textures of foods like chips and ice cream to ensure people will want to eat more.

ACCESS AND AFFORDABILITY

One report found that the lowest income populations spent 36 percent more of their income on food when compared to the highest income populations who spent just 8 percent on food. US consumers spend an average of 8.6 percent of their income on food, but as incomes rise, money spent on food represents a smaller portion of the budget. Studies show that low-income individuals and those using public programs like SNAP spend and intake more sweets and salty snacks. Millions also live in "food deserts," or areas with limited access to supermarkets or grocery stores that can make it harder to eat a healthy diet. Easier access to fast food, including takeout delivery, can be more tempting than cooking at home (see pages 46–47). Obesity prevalence is much higher in low-income children and adolescents than in higher income groups with nearly 19 percent and 11 percent, respectively. With higher rates of obesity comes diet-related disease that may impact their quality of life.

Learn to say "No"

HAVE YOU EVER ACCEPTED AN EXTRA HELPING EVEN THOUGH YOU WERE FULL?
We seem to be susceptible to eating more with others than alone, although the underlying reasons aren't clear. Some "social facilitation" studies show eating with friends and family in particular can increase intake; this could be because chatting with others distracts attention from food, or eating a greater amount is more acceptable in larger groups. A research review suggests meals eaten socially could be a third to a half bigger.

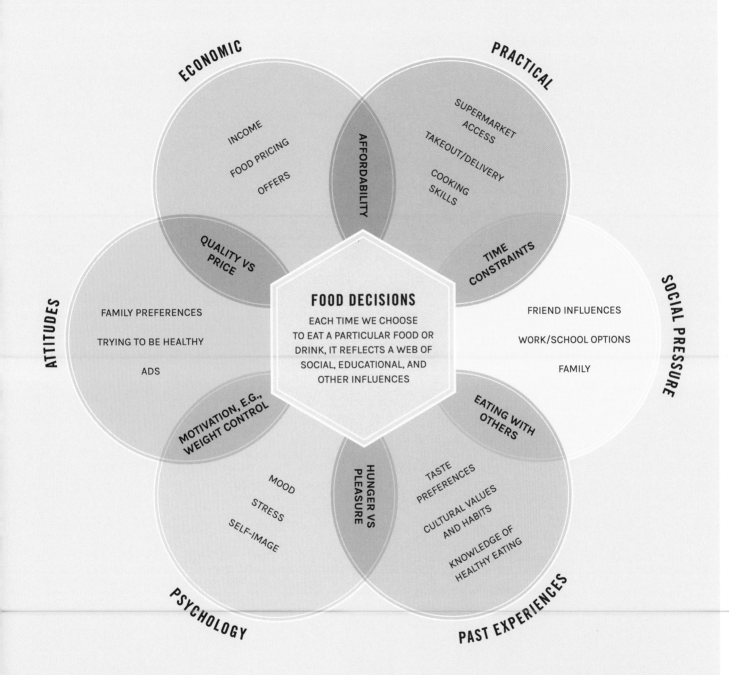

ECONOMIC

PRACTICAL

SOCIAL PRESSURE

PAST EXPERIENCES

PSYCHOLOGY

ATTITUDES

INCOME

FOOD PRICING

OFFERS

AFFORDABILITY

SUPERMARKET ACCESS

TAKEOUT/DELIVERY

COOKING SKILLS

TIME CONSTRAINTS

QUALITY VS PRICE

FAMILY PREFERENCES

TRYING TO BE HEALTHY

ADS

FOOD DECISIONS

EACH TIME WE CHOOSE TO EAT A PARTICULAR FOOD OR DRINK, IT REFLECTS A WEB OF SOCIAL, EDUCATIONAL, AND OTHER INFLUENCES

FRIEND INFLUENCES

WORK/SCHOOL OPTIONS

FAMILY

EATING WITH OTHERS

MOTIVATION, E.G., WEIGHT CONTROL

HUNGER VS PLEASURE

MOOD

STRESS

SELF-IMAGE

TASTE PREFERENCES

CULTURAL VALUES AND HABITS

KNOWLEDGE OF HEALTHY EATING

SHOULD I AVOID PROCESSED FOOD?

There are good reasons why processed food is a large part of the modern diet—
it's often cheaper than fresh, allows for a huge amount of choice, and is convenient.
But not all processed food is equal, and it's important to understand the differences.

Processed food isn't automatically inferior or unhealthy compared to fresh. Some nutrient-rich whole foods like vegetables, fish, milk, or whole grains are processed simply for storage or preservation; for example, freezing happens straight after harvest, so freshly picked foods arrive in stores at near peak nutritional value.

Likewise, canning is processing but retains much of the protein of fish and the fiber of fruits and vegetables. However, skinless fruit in syrup has less fiber and more sugar than whole fruit; choose fruit in water, or discard the syrup, or beans in water rather than sauce or brine.

Certain processed foods have been altered for flavor or texture or have additives to extend shelf life; even so, foods like whole wheat bread, rolled oats, sauerkraut, and tomato paste still fit easily into healthy eating. Some are fortified to replace vitamins or minerals lost during processing or to boost nutrients for plant-based eaters.

HIGHLY PROCESSED FOODS

These should be limited in a healthy, balanced diet. They typically combine already modified ingredients and additives and are either ready to eat or need minimal preparation; examples include many sweets, chips, baked goods, and ready meals. They lack much of the original whole food's fiber, making them easily digestible, while added salt, sugar, and fats also make them highly palatable. The mechanisms behind their suggested addictive nature include sugar's ability to stimulate the brain's reward centers.

In the US, nearly 60 percent of average daily energy intake is now said to come from highly processed foods; evidence suggests rising sales and obesity rates are associated (although obesity has many causes). For example, high-fructose corn syrup is a type of sugar widely added to highly processed foods in the US; since the body has no biochemical reactions that use it, excess is turned into fat in the liver.

Degrees of processing

Any food you buy in a supermarket will have undergone some form of processing, but the impact on its nutritional value can vary widely. Corn, for example, can be eaten in a range of different forms, including as a refined ingredient in highly processed foods.

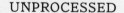

UNPROCESSED

Fresh sweet corn
This is still in its natural state, although it may have been cleaned prior to sale.

MINIMALLY PROCESSED

Canned sweet corn
Canned vegetables usually retain fiber; salt may be added for preservation.

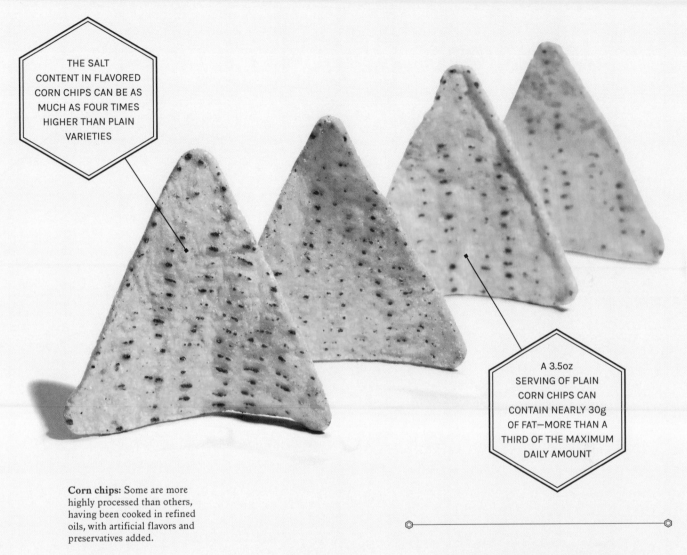

THE SALT CONTENT IN FLAVORED CORN CHIPS CAN BE AS MUCH AS FOUR TIMES HIGHER THAN PLAIN VARIETIES

A 3.5oz SERVING OF PLAIN CORN CHIPS CAN CONTAIN NEARLY 30g OF FAT—MORE THAN A THIRD OF THE MAXIMUM DAILY AMOUNT

Corn chips: Some are more highly processed than others, having been cooked in refined oils, with artificial flavors and preservatives added.

PROCESSED

Popcorn
It has been altered but may be freshly made simply by heat, or may contain additives, fat, salt, or sugar.

HIGHLY PROCESSED

High-fructose corn syrup
This is made from cornstarch and is often used as a sweetener in the US.

Are additives bad?

ADDITIVES ARE OFTEN USED IN PROCESSED FOODS TO IMITATE NATURAL FLAVORS, MAKE FOOD FEEL BETTER IN THE MOUTH, OR AID WITH PROCESSING. They can be synthetic or naturally derived, like ascorbic acid, which is vitamin C. Monosodium glutamate (MSG) is a widely used flavor enhancer. While there is a lack of evidence on its long-term effects on health, some studies have suggested a link with obesity, central nervous system disorders, and liver damage. Additives are rigorously tested and deemed safe for use; if you have concerns, check labels and reduce your intake.

SHOULD I PAY ATTENTION TO FOOD LABELS?

Nutritional information on food packaging can appear confusing at first. But it's not too difficult to decode the data, and understanding it will let you make more informed choices about your daily diet.

Checking the nutrition panel on food packaging can, for example, help you spot that a low-fat yogurt has had extra sugar added, making a higher-fat option with less sugar a smarter choice. Rules around nutritional labeling vary in different countries; in the US, most prepackaged foods must show the following per serving:

- Energy in kilocalories or calories
- Total and saturated fats
- Protein
- Total carbohydrates from sugars that are added and naturally present
- Salt, which may also be listed as "sodium"

The nutrition label must show the number of servings per package and may also show nutritional information per entire package. Manufacturers can choose whether to show information about vitamins, minerals, dietary fiber, and certain nutrients.

HEALTH CLAIMS

Health, nutrient content, and structure/function claims are useful for making a quick decision about a product and comparing similar items. They aren't mandatory, and some show only the amount of energy (calories), but they visually display whether the food is low, medium, or high in salt, sugar, and saturated fat. The numbers tell you how much of each is in a portion, both in grams and as a share of the total daily recommended amount. Food suppliers can decide on the portion size shown on the label, which could be less than what's inside the package—so if you eat extra, you'll consume more than it says.

Facts Up Front

THIS US VOLUNTARY LABEL IDEA WAS DEVELOPED BY FOOD INDUSTRY BODIES. Labels show the amount of calories and nutrients to limit in a standardized serving amount, like a cup. The label can highlight up to two "positive" components, like a specific vitamin.

PER 1 CUP SERVING

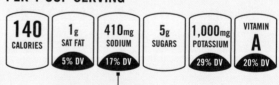

| 140 CALORIES | 1g SAT FAT 5% DV | 410mg SODIUM 17% DV | 5g SUGARS | 1,000mg POTASSIUM 29% DV | VITAMIN A 20% DV |

Percentage of daily allowance

Monitor your sugar, fat, and salt

Sugar, saturated fat, and salt intake should be controlled as part of healthy eating. Use these steps to become more aware of how much you eat in each meal or snack and over a whole day.

1.

KNOW THE DAILY MAXIMUM

These are the maximum daily intake amounts in US health guidelines. (They are based on an average woman, in terms of body size and activity levels, so they will vary, for instance, for a highly active man.)

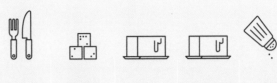

CALORIES	ADDED SUGAR	TOTAL FAT	SATURATED FAT	SALT
2,000	<50g	<77g	<22g	<2,000 mg

2.

CALCULATE BY WEIGHT

The nutrition panel on packaging lists sugar, fat, and salt per serving; figure out the total amounts in the food and check whether they fit into your daily amounts.

KEY

- High
- Medium
- Low

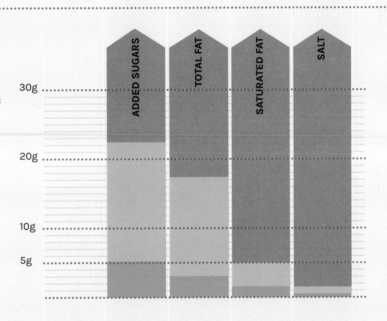

3.

CHECK BY SERVING

Labels help you assess the sugar, salt, and fat in one serving/portion and track how your intake is adding up.

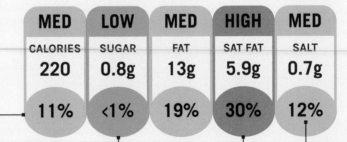

MED	LOW	MED	HIGH	MED
CALORIES	SUGAR	FAT	SAT FAT	SALT
220	0.8g	13g	5.9g	0.7g
11%	<1%	19%	30%	12%

Amber: More of these indicate the food can be eaten regularly

Green: The more of these there are on the label, the healthier a choice it is

Red: You may want to eat a small amount, have it occasionally, or choose an alternative

Check %daily values: These show how much a serving contributes to the maximum daily amount

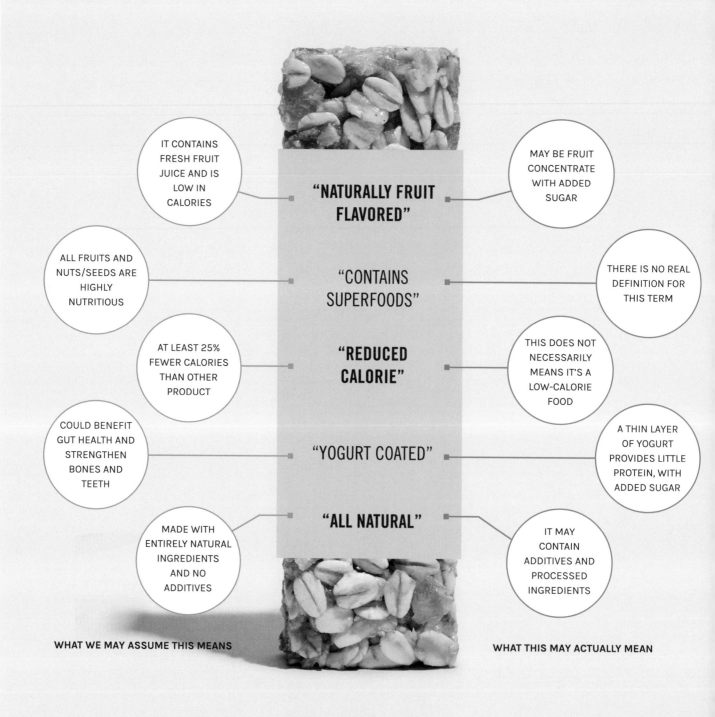

"NATURALLY FRUIT FLAVORED"

IT CONTAINS FRESH FRUIT JUICE AND IS LOW IN CALORIES

MAY BE FRUIT CONCENTRATE WITH ADDED SUGAR

"CONTAINS SUPERFOODS"

ALL FRUITS AND NUTS/SEEDS ARE HIGHLY NUTRITIOUS

THERE IS NO REAL DEFINITION FOR THIS TERM

"REDUCED CALORIE"

AT LEAST 25% FEWER CALORIES THAN OTHER PRODUCT

THIS DOES NOT NECESSARILY MEANS IT'S A LOW-CALORIE FOOD

"YOGURT COATED"

COULD BENEFIT GUT HEALTH AND STRENGTHEN BONES AND TEETH

A THIN LAYER OF YOGURT PROVIDES LITTLE PROTEIN, WITH ADDED SUGAR

"ALL NATURAL"

MADE WITH ENTIRELY NATURAL INGREDIENTS AND NO ADDITIVES

IT MAY CONTAIN ADDITIVES AND PROCESSED INGREDIENTS

WHAT WE MAY ASSUME THIS MEANS

WHAT THIS MAY ACTUALLY MEAN

Messages on foods often emphasize them as a healthy choice; while some ingredients may be, the overall nutritional value may not match our perceptions.

CAN I TRUST MARKETING BUZZWORDS?

Food manufacturers and suppliers spend huge amounts on crafting messages that influence our perceptions about nutritional value, to entice us to choose their particular product. Don't take these at face value.

Claims on food packaging can be about health, nutritional content, or structure/function and are regulated by the FDA. To be FDA approved, the claim must be supported by the totality of publicly available scientific evidence. A US study found that highlighting added vitamins in snacks made consumers more likely to view them as healthier and less likely to check the nutrition label.

NO ADDED SUGAR

"Sugar free" means one serving contains less than 0.5g of sugar, both natural and added. "No added sugar" refers only to sugars added during processing, not naturally occurring sugar, such as fructose in fruit. A no-added-sugar fruit smoothie, for example, could potentially contain more sugar than a can of soda.

LOW/LIGHT

The claim "low" refers to the following amounts compared to a given reference amount: <40 calories; <3g total fat; <1g saturated fat (with no more than 15% of calories coming from saturated fat); <140mg sodium; and <20mg cholesterol (and only when a food contains <2g of saturated fat per serving). Food that derives less than 50% of its calories from fat can be labeled "light" or "lite" if its total amount of calories is decreased by at least 33.3% or its fat content is reduced by at least 50% compared to a standard/original version.

HIGH FIBER

Food products that contain at least 10% DV or 2.5g of fiber per serving can claim they are a "good source of fiber," and those containing at least 20% DV of fiber or 5g or more of fiber per serving can label the product with a high fiber claim.

NATURAL/ORGANIC

The FDA defines "natural" as having nothing artificial or synthetic (including all color additives) included in or added to the food. The claim "100% organic" can appear on any product that contains 100% organic ingredients (excluding salt and water).

GOOD SOURCE/EXCELLENT SOURCE

If a food contains 10–19% DV of a certain nutrient, it's considered a "good source." An "excellent source" has at least 20% DV of a certain nutrient.

Unhealthy influence

SOCIAL MEDIA IS A MATRIX OF MISINFORMATION AND PSEUDOSCIENTIFIC CLAIMS.
For example, nearly half of social media users reportedly think cutting out a whole food group is healthy. A study of nine popular UK influencers blogging about weight management found that only two had relevant qualifications, and five didn't cite evidence-based references for nutrition claims. Influencers often have a commercial agenda—be wary of their recommendations around food.

IS SUGAR THE ENEMY?

Although sugar has been regarded the enemy for a long while, the truth is that not all sugars are bad for us. Sugar has its place in the diet—in the right quantities and in a form your body can handle comfortably.

Sugar is a carbohydrate found in many foods (see pages 12–13). Foods containing natural sugars, such as fruits and dairy products, are good sources of many nutrients and the energy provided by sugar.

Despite its bad reputation, scientists have not proved that sugar affects health when it is not part of a diet too high in calories.

ADDED SUGARS

Added sugar might be sugar added to an oat bar during production or a spoonful of honey in herbal tea.

Foods containing added sugars often have little or no nutritional benefit. The World Health Organization (WHO) recommends no more than 5 percent of daily energy intake comes from added sugars.

Sugars, often chemically produced, are added to products to enhance palatability. Check sugar content on labels (see pages 60–61). It may be referred to as "total sugars," which includes naturally occurring and added sugars. Sugar comes in many forms—sucrose, glucose, fructose, maltose, fruit juice, molasses, corn and other syrups, honey, and fruit juice concentrate.

Avoid high-fructose corn syrup (HFCS), which is packaged into many foods in the US. Countries consuming HFCS the most show higher levels of diabetes. It has been shown that a diet of more than 150g per day of HFCS reduces insulin sensitivity (see page 172), increasing the risk of developing high blood pressure and high cholesterol levels.

THE RIGHT BALANCE

Science confirms what we all know—sugar affects the feel-good reward center in the brain. It triggers a pleasure response that's similar to how we feel when watching cute puppies or receiving love. Perhaps that explains why sugar provides more calories in

---

Added and "free" sugars

While not an added sugar, fruit juice is an example of a "free" sugar. Once the sugar it contains is separated from the fruit's pulp, the fiber (and bulk) is lost. You wouldn't eat four oranges in one sitting, but you might drink their juice in one large glass of orange juice—which is more sugar than you'd find in a can of soda!

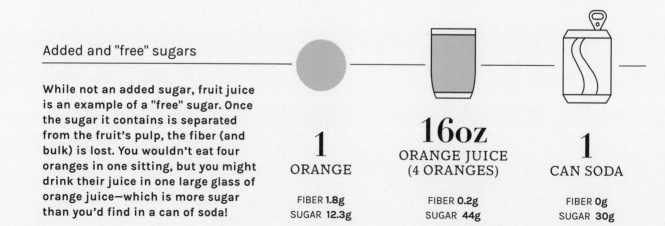

1
ORANGE

FIBER **1.8g**
SUGAR **12.3g**

16oz
ORANGE JUICE
(4 ORANGES)

FIBER **0.2g**
SUGAR **44g**

1
CAN SODA

FIBER **0g**
SUGAR **30g**

our diets than is advisable. But there's no need to demonize it. Psychology plays a major role in the nutrition choices we make. Going teetotal on any food may lead to binging; moderation is best.

REDUCING SUGAR

Ensure you're aware of how much sugar you are consuming, so you can make appropriate choices to help you stay within the recommended allowance.

Swap out sugary foods for alternatives. Substitute cookies, and add fruit instead of sugar to breakfast cereals, for instance.

Have smaller portions. Share dessert with a loved one. Ask for sugar-laden dressings on the side so you can use less. Condiments like ketchup can have 23g of sugar per 100g; use 1 teaspoon per serving. When cooking, don't add sugar to savory foods.

Nearly a quarter of the added sugar in our diets comes from sugar-sweetened beverages (fizzy drinks, sweetened juices, and fruit-flavored beverages). Swap sugary drinks for water.

It may take time to settle into your new habits, but there is no conclusive research linking sugar with physical addiction in humans. You can't experience withdrawal symptoms as you would with a dependency on alcohol or drugs.

Sugar alternatives

IF YOU DRINK MANY SUGAR-SWEETENED BEVERAGES, CONSIDER USING SWEETENERS TO HELP YOU GRADUALLY WEAN YOURSELF OFF ADDING SUGAR TO TEA OR COFFEE.
Molasses, maple syrup, and honey come from natural sources. Artificial sweeteners, such as sucralose, aspartame, and saccharine, are chemically manufactured. Both natural and artificial sweeteners are safe to use in moderation. There is some research suggesting that the latter are not beneficial to the gut microbiome, but as this is a relatively new field of research, the evidence is not conclusive.

Recommended allowance
The American Heart Association recommends limiting sugar to 6 teaspoons or 100 calories per day for women, and about 9 teaspoons or 150 calories per day for men.

6–9
SUGAR CUBES OR TEASPOONS IS THE RECOMMENDED DAILY ALLOWANCE OF SUGARS

IS FAT STILL BAD FOR ME?

Scientific thinking on fat has shifted dramatically in recent decades, and it's a complex area that is still developing today. However, there is general agreement that we should all enjoy some healthier fats within our diet.

Fat is actually crucial to our well-being. It gives us energy, delivers flavor to food, and helps us feel full and satisfied. The body requires fat to absorb certain vitamins. We should try to include both mono- and polyunsaturated fats, particularly omega-3 fatty acids, which come only from diet and are proven to help lower LDL (low-density lipoprotein) cholesterol and support heart health and cognition.

ARE THERE "BAD" FATS?

Research has discredited the broad "fat is bad" viewpoint that led to a proliferation of low-fat diet plans and foods. A 2017 study explored reduced-fat diets over eight years and found no noticeable health benefits over diets that didn't restrict fat; one possible factor may be eating the extra sugar often added by manufacturers to replace lost flavor.

Trans fats, or artificially hardened vegetable oils, are banned in several countries, including the US, due to concerns they raise LDL cholesterol, a cause of heart disease and stroke. They are used rarely in UK foods, at very low levels—look for "partially hydrogenated" on labels. Saturated fat is found mainly in animal-derived foods and cereal products like pizza and cookies. There is evidence that a high intake of saturated fat raises LDL cholesterol.

Recently, scientific debate has emerged over the link between saturated fat and heart disease, with one research review suggesting that saturated fat doesn't raise the risk of heart disease. However, the American and British Heart associations advise that replacing saturated fat with unsaturated lowers the risk, and health bodies, including the World Health Organization, advise limiting saturated fat to no more than 10%–11% of daily calories. Most experts agree that a healthy diet will do more to reduce heart disease risk than focusing on saturated fat. The key is to eat less food that's high in saturated fat and replace it with healthier fats from fish and plants—not added sugars or refined carbohydrates.

Which fat is healthiest?

Oils and fats contain different combinations of unsaturated and saturated fatty acids per 100g, making some a healthier choice. Their versatility for cooking depends on their smoke points—the temperature range at which they degrade and may release potentially harmful compounds.

EXTRA-VIRGIN OLIVE OIL

SATURATED FAT: **15.5g**
POLYUNSATURATED FAT: **10.7g**
MONOUNSATURATED FAT: **65g**
SMOKE POINT: **374°F–405°F**

Good for heart health, this oil is more suited to lower-temperature cooking, dressing, or marinating.

CANOLA OIL

SATURATED FAT: **6g**
POLYUNSATURATED FAT: **27g**
MONOUNSATURATED FAT: **54g**
SMOKE POINT: **400°F–446°F**

Its combination of unsaturated fats make this is a good choice for a heart-healthy daily cooking oil; it can be used for frying and roasting.

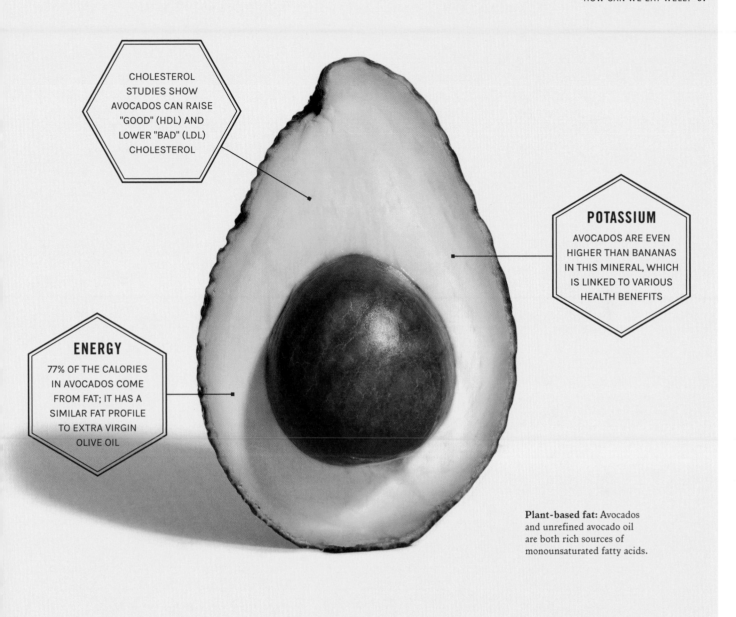

CHOLESTEROL
STUDIES SHOW
AVOCADOS CAN RAISE
"GOOD" (HDL) AND
LOWER "BAD" (LDL)
CHOLESTEROL

POTASSIUM
AVOCADOS ARE EVEN
HIGHER THAN BANANAS
IN THIS MINERAL, WHICH
IS LINKED TO VARIOUS
HEALTH BENEFITS

ENERGY
77% OF THE CALORIES
IN AVOCADOS COME
FROM FAT; IT HAS A
SIMILAR FAT PROFILE
TO EXTRA VIRGIN
OLIVE OIL

Plant-based fat: Avocados
and unrefined avocado oil
are both rich sources of
monounsaturated fatty acids.

SUNFLOWER OIL

SATURATED FAT: **10g**
POLYUNSATURATED FAT: **56g**
MONOUNSATURATED FAT: **25.8g**
SMOKE POINT: **446°F**

Widely used for cooking, it contains a
high level of omega-6 fatty acids, which
can help reduce cholesterol but have
also been linked to inflammation.

COCONUT OIL

SATURATED FAT: **86.5g**
POLYUNSATURATED FAT: **1.8g**
MONOUNSATURATED FAT: **5.8g**
SMOKE POINT: **347°F–385°F**

This plant oil contains mostly
saturated fatty acids and has been
found to raise LDL cholesterol so is
best used occasionally.

BUTTER

SATURATED FAT: **67g**
POLYUNSATURATED FAT: **5g**
MONOUNSATURATED FAT: **28g**
SMOKE POINT: **300°F–347°F**

Butter is primarily a saturated fat
but is also a source of vitamins
A and D and contains calcium.

SHOULD I CUT OUT RED MEAT?

We know that consuming different kinds of protein—including plants, fish, and poultry—is a sensible step toward healthy eating. But if you really enjoy things like steaks and hot dogs, consider their nutritional and health implications.

Red meat is red when raw and includes lamb, beef, venison, pork, and veal. It's a rich source of muscle-building protein and important micronutrients, notably vitamins B3 and B12 (not available from plants), iron, zinc, and selenium. While it's nutritious, it can be high in saturated fat, especially fattier cuts; 3.5oz of prime rib contains around 34g of total fat. One limited study found organic meat contains 50 percent more omega-3 fatty acids, known to support the heart and immune system, possibly because livestock eat a more grass-based diet.

Processed meats like ham, bacon, and salami have been cured, salted, smoked, or otherwise altered to improve flavor and for longer life and often contain a lot of salt. A diet high in salt and saturated fat has been shown to raise blood pressure and LDL cholesterol, a risk factor for cardiovascular disease.

CANCER RISK

The pigment in fresh red meat, called heme, and nitrite or nitrate preservatives used in processing have both been linked to increased bowel cancer risk. Although nitrites also occur naturally in green vegetables, the way the body digests them in meat can create toxic nitrosamines. In 2015, World Health Organization cancer experts identified red meat as a probable cause of cancers and processed meats a definite cause (although not how many cases they cause). However, not all processed meat products contain nitrites; for example, traditionally produced *prosciutto di Parma* is cured with salt.

One recent US study concluded that evidence didn't support eating less red or processed meat, but this was challenged by several health bodies. The World Cancer Research Fund advises adults to eat little or no processed meat and up to 12oz–18oz cooked weight of red meat weekly, while some guidelines suggest regular consumers eat no more than 3oz in total a day. A more recent finding concluded that eating 3oz daily—about three slices of ham—could still elevate cancer risk, although overall diet and lifestyle matters, too. If you eat red meat, opt for unprocessed, lean cuts with plenty of vegetables.

What's in your sausage?

NOT ALL SAUSAGES ARE NUTRITIONALLY EQUAL IN TERMS OF MEAT, SALT, AND FAT CONTENT.
For example, a survey found salt in premade sausages varied from 0.75g to 2.3g per 3.5oz. Freshly made sausages or burgers may be a healthier choice and may not be a cancer risk unless they are further modified—ask your butcher what's in them. One research review noted the link between colorectal cancers and sodium nitrite but claimed this isn't added to most traditional sausages.

Cooking fresh or processed meat

Cooking can create substances called HCAs and PAHs that are mutagenic; they can be activated by enzymes during digestion and cause DNA changes that may increase cancer risk.

FRESH MEAT

PROCESSED MEAT

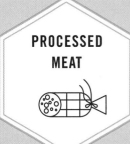

+ **+**

HIGH HEAT

$390^{0}F+$

PAN FRYING, GRILLING & ROASTING

BARBECUING

HCAs

When meat, poultry, or fish cooks at high temperature, especially if it's overcooked, creatine in muscle and amino acids can react and form HCAs (heterocyclic amines).

PAHs

Fat from meat grilled at high heat can drip onto an open fire, creating smoke containing PAHs (polycyclic aromatic hydrocarbons) that can stick to the meat's surface; PAHs can also form when meat is smoked.

NITROSAMINES

Nitrosamine molecules are present in some processed meats and are probable human carcinogens; research has found higher levels in bacon that has been fried.

MARINATING MEAT
IN OLIVE OIL, LEMON JUICE, OR RED WINE CAN REDUCE HCAs BY UP TO

90%

CHARRING
INDICATES THAT PAHs MAY BE PRESENT; AVOID EATING THE MEAT OR SCRAPE BURNT AREAS

KEY

➡ Fresh meat

➡ Processed meat

WILL SALT GIVE ME A HEART ATTACK?

If you like to add salt to your meals but you've never thought much about the salt content that's in so many everyday foods, from baked beans to cookies, there is a chance your eating habits could be harming your health.

Salt is partly made of sodium, and our bodies need some sodium for biological processes like fluid regulation and nerve impulse transmission. But research estimates that US adults consume an average 3,400mg of salt a day; the US guideline daily limit is 2,300mg—about a teaspoon.

For decades, the consensus among leading health bodies and experts, including the World Health Organization (WHO), has been that eating too much sodium can lead to high blood pressure, a major risk factor for stroke, kidney disease, and cardiovascular disease, which can lead to heart attack.

In 2018, an international study gained headlines for concluding that this risk would require a significantly higher average salt intake than most people actually eat (China being an exception), but the basis of the research was challenged. The WHO continues to advise adults to restrict salt intake to 5g (5,000mg) a day.

ARE PREMIUM SALTS HEALTHIER?

Sea salt crystals and flakes and coarse mined rock salt like Himalayan pink salt are less refined than table salt, which has minerals removed as it is finely ground and anti-caking agents are added.

Brain

Heart

Kidneys

Salt and hypertension

High blood pressure (hypertension) caused by a long-term diet high in salt could potentially damage the heart, brain, and other organs.

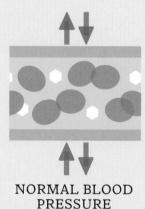

NORMAL BLOOD PRESSURE

Artery walls expand and contract as the heart pumps to circulate blood.

Although one survey found that nearly two-thirds of people think sea salt contains less sodium, the American Heart Association says table salt and most sea salts are around 40 percent sodium by weight, and there are no health reasons for choosing sea salt.

"HIDDEN" SALT

Many people don't realize they are eating too much salt because around 75 percent of the salt in our diet is already in processed and prepreparedfoods. It's no surprise foods like soy sauce, processed meats, and many snacks and ready-made meals are high in salt. But it's also present in foods you might not expect, like cookies and cakes, and those you may eat regularly, like bread and cereals. Even vegetables

can be high in salt when canned in brine—if you can't buy fresh veggies, it may be better to choose frozen because salt isn't used during freezing.

Salt content in similar products can vary, so check labels. These may list salt or sodium; multiply sodium by 2.5 to get the salt content.

REDUCING SALT:

● Aim to reduce salt gradually—our taste buds get used to salt intake, so it should get easier over time. Check food labels and opt for products containing less salt where possible.

● Experiment with herbs and spices for flavor; keep plenty of dried options handy.

● In restaurants, ask for your meal to be prepared without added salt.

SALT INTAKE

US GUIDELINES SUGGEST DAILY MAXIMUMS OF:

AGE 0–6 mths
<**110mg**

AGE 7–12 mths
<**370mg**

AGE 1–3 years
<**1,500mg**

AGE 4–8 years
<**1,900mg**

AGE 14+
<**2,300mg**

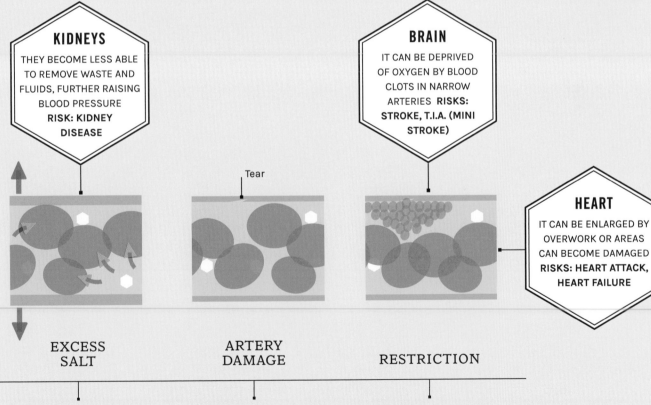

KIDNEYS
THEY BECOME LESS ABLE TO REMOVE WASTE AND FLUIDS, FURTHER RAISING BLOOD PRESSURE **RISK: KIDNEY DISEASE**

BRAIN
IT CAN BE DEPRIVED OF OXYGEN BY BLOOD CLOTS IN NARROW ARTERIES **RISKS: STROKE, T.I.A. (MINI STROKE)**

HEART
IT CAN BE ENLARGED BY OVERWORK OR AREAS CAN BECOME DAMAGED **RISKS: HEART ATTACK, HEART FAILURE**

Tear

EXCESS SALT

ARTERY DAMAGE

RESTRICTION

The body reacts to excess salt by retaining water in the blood, increasing blood volume and pressure on arteries.

Pressure can eventually cause artery walls to narrow, tear, and stiffen, reducing blood flow.

Artery damage makes it easier for cholesterol to collect there, leading to blockages that can restrict oxygen.

SURELY CAFFEINE CAN'T BE GOOD FOR ME?

Caffeine is the world's most commonly consumed psychoactive substance, but is it okay to have as much as you like?

————

Caffeine occurs naturally in coffee, cocoa, and tea plants and is added to some drinks, food, and medications. It boosts alertness by stimulating the central nervous system and blocking adenosine, a molecule that reduces heart rate and promotes sleep.

Moderate caffeine intake—around 300mg–400mg per day, or 3–4 cups of coffee—can have beneficial effects, including a reduced risk of heart disease and enhanced concentration. Many studies show that caffeine aids athletic performance, for instance, by boosting metabolic rate and glycogen (fuel) storage if taken prior to high-intensity interval training. Research (albeit not as strong) also suggests caffeine may help relieve headaches and migraines. Most studies are based on coffee, which also contains antioxidants and potassium, a mineral that has been shown to help lower blood pressure.

CAN I HAVE TOO MUCH?

More than 600mg of caffeine daily can cause anxiety, upset stomach, and raised blood pressure; frequent consumption may worsen irritable bowel syndrome symptoms. If taken less than six hours before bed, caffeine can disrupt sleep; it may also stimulate a need to urinate. Pregnant women should limit intake to 200mg daily, due to an association with low birth weight and miscarriage. Despite some scientific debate on the issue, the World Health Organization recognizes caffeine addiction as a clinical disorder. Reactions to caffeine vary, but many can safely enjoy moderate consumption.

Adrenaline rush: Consuming caffeine increases brain activity, prompting the release of adrenaline and a series of "fight-or-flight" effects.

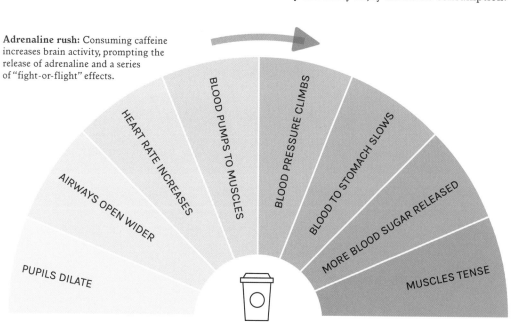

PUPILS DILATE

AIRWAYS OPEN WIDER

HEART RATE INCREASES

BLOOD PUMPS TO MUSCLES

BLOOD PRESSURE CLIMBS

BLOOD TO STOMACH SLOWS

MORE BLOOD SUGAR RELEASED

MUSCLES TENSE

CAFFEINE SOURCES

CAFFEINE IS FOUND IN MANY PRODUCTS. THESE ARE SOME TYPICAL AMOUNTS IN MILLIGRAMS (mg).

95 – 125

Coffee
8oz (240ml)

91

Energy drink
8oz (240ml)

42

Diet cola
11oz (330ml)

26

Black tea
8oz (240ml)

16

Dark chocolate
1oz (20g)

DOES ALCOHOL HAVE ANY BENEFITS?

While moderate alcohol intake may have some positive health impacts, the risks of drinking in excess are well established.

Alcohol has no nutritional benefits that warrant introducing it. Several studies have associated moderate consumption of any alcohol with lower risk of coronary heart disease; however, definitions of "moderate" vary.

Red wine can contain organic compounds called polyphenols; their antioxidant and anti-inflammatory properties may have preventive and/or therapeutic effects for cardiovascular disease, neurodegenerative disorders, cancer, and obesity. Red wine has around 10 times more polyphenols than white. Comparisons show lower incidences of heart disease in wine-drinking countries like France compared to those with a higher intake of beer or spirits, such as Germany and Russia (although wine-drinking countries often have healthier diets, and this is based on moderate consumption).

MAXIMUM AMOUNTS

The US's recommended alcohol intake is one drink or less per day for women and two drinks or less per day for men (on days when alcohol is consumed). One alcohol drink is equivalent to 12oz of regular beer, 5oz of wine, or 1.5oz of 80-proof distilled spirits.

Heavier, and prolonged, drinking can lead to health problems, including increased blood pressure, heart disease, liver disease, and depression. Alcohol also stimulates appetite, and one survey suggested that 80 percent of people are not aware of the calories in a glass of wine.

Drinking patterns also matter. A study found consuming around one drink daily across four or more days a week resulted in lower death rates than the same amount over 1–2 days. To reduce intake, aim for several alcohol-free days a week.

Calories in alcohol: Spirits tend to have fewest calories per serving, without mixers.

61

Rum
Single
(1oz/25ml)

110

Vodka
Single
(1oz/25ml)

61+93

Gin & tonic
Single (1oz/25ml
+ 5oz/150ml)

160

Red wine
1 glass
(6oz/175ml)

182

Beer/pale ale
1 pint
(16oz)

216

Cider
1 pint
(16oz)

WILL SUPERFOODS SAVE ME?

So-called "superfoods" seem to be everywhere, from social media to supermarket shelves, with new arrivals constantly being talked about. Are these foods all hype or healthy enough to earn our attention—and their price?

No single food can compensate for an unhealthy diet or prevent illness. So-called "superfoods" supposedly offer a particular health benefit or promote wellness—in fact, this is a marketing term to entice us into buying more of various exotic-sounding foods. It appears to work: in 2015 alone, the number of new products labeled "superfood," "supergrain," or "superfruit" rose by a third.

Foods often called "super," like spirulina and goji berries, can pack a nutritional punch—3.5oz of dried goji berries contains 4mg of vitamin A, compared to 2.5mg in fresh carrots. Research suggests their mix of phytochemicals and high nutrient levels can help improve overall health, support the immune system, regulate mood by increasing serotonin, and more. However, a lot of this comes from animal studies.

It's also worth noting that we can absorb only a certain amount of any nutrient. Even supposed superfoods are beneficial only when consumed in moderation, as part of a balanced diet; for example, turmeric and curcumin can increase bile secretion. Check with your doctor before consuming.

COST OF "SUPERFOODS"

These foods are often more expensive than common fruits and vegetables with similar nutritional benefits. For example, 3.5oz of papaya contains 61mg of vitamin C, compared to 77.6mg in bell peppers, while a cup of whole milk has significantly more calcium than 3.5oz of spirulina. Although goji berries have more vitamin A than carrots by weight, over a week, you're likely to eat more carrots—and so take in as much, if not more, vitamin A at less cost. At the time of writing, in one supermarket, goji berries were 40 times more expensive than carrots per 3.5oz.

In addition to expense, foods like goji berries, açai, spirulina, and chia may be hard to find. Buying more readily available alternatives could help offset some of the environmental concerns around importing foods from around the globe.

CHIA SEEDS

If eaten in the right amount and within a healthy diet, these are a source of fiber, calcium, and phosphorus.

ALTERNATIVE
FLAXSEEDS
SESAME SEEDS

SPIRULINA

Including omega-3 and -6 fatty acids and iron, this algae is said to have antioxidant and anti-inflammatory properties.

ALTERNATIVE
WHOLE MILK

AÇAI

Usually sold frozen or powdered due to their short life span, these berries contain antioxidants and fiber.

ALTERNATIVE
BLUEBERRIES
CRANBERRIES

GINGER

Ginger is thought to have anti-inflammatory and antioxidant effects, although research is limited.

ALTERNATIVE
N/A

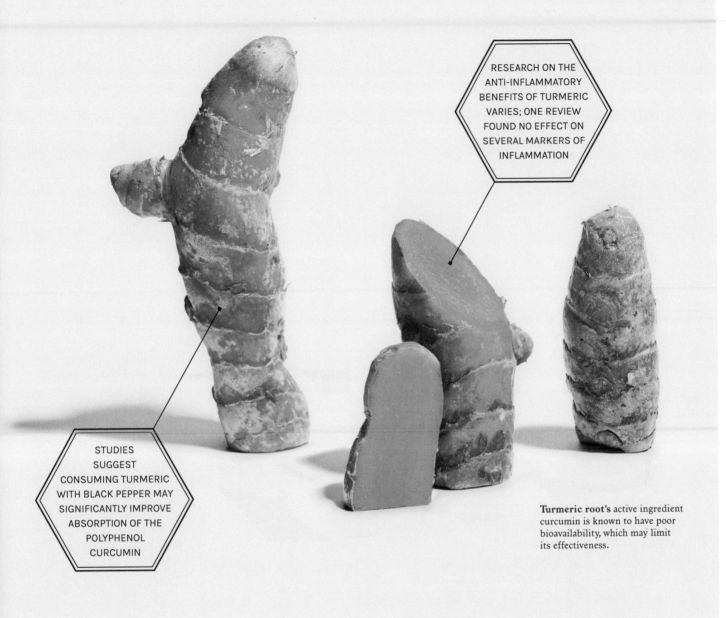

RESEARCH ON THE
ANTI-INFLAMMATORY
BENEFITS OF TURMERIC
VARIES; ONE REVIEW
FOUND NO EFFECT ON
SEVERAL MARKERS OF
INFLAMMATION

STUDIES
SUGGEST
CONSUMING TURMERIC
WITH BLACK PEPPER MAY
SIGNIFICANTLY IMPROVE
ABSORPTION OF THE
POLYPHENOL
CURCUMIN

Turmeric root's active ingredient curcumin is known to have poor bioavailability, which may limit its effectiveness.

GOJI BERRIES

These are rich in carotenoids, which act as antioxidants, and have benefits relating to vision and macular degeneration.

ALTERNATIVE
SWEET POTATO
CARROTS

AVOCADO

This fruit is a source of monounsaturated fatty acids (linked to blood cholesterol benefits), vitamin E, and fiber.

ALTERNATIVE
BANANAS

PAPAYA

Research suggests its antioxidant carotenoids, in particular lycopene, are particularly well absorbed.

ALTERNATIVE
BELL PEPPERS

TURMERIC

Often consumed as powder, it contains the polyphenol curcumin, which may have anti-inflammatory effects.

ALTERNATIVE
N/A

IS ORGANIC BETTER FOR YOU?

Many people now think organic food is safer, healthier, and tastier than regular food. Others say it's better for the environment and improves animal welfare. You can pay up to 200 percent more for an organic label, but is it all marketing hype?

The focus of organic production is usually based on environmental sustainability and human well-being. It is easy to see how organic is perceived as healthier, the image of wildlife and nature untouched by mankind, it can paint a very vivid picture in our imaginations of the way we want to see the food we eat in harmony with the world.

People are willing to pay more for this ideal. Organic food comes with a price tag, so while the more privileged among us may be able to shop organic, for many people, it is simply not an option.

THE EVIDENCE ON ORGANIC

While there may be respected studies that find more nutrients in organic foods, a great many others have found insufficient evidence to recommend organic over nonorganic for health or safety. One review of 233 studies concluded that there is no strong evidence to suggest that organic foods are significantly more nutritious than conventionally farmed foods. This was also the conclusion of the UK Food Standards Agency (FSA), though their research considered just 11 studies. (The FSA publicly supports consumer choice and is not pro- or anti-organic food.)

There are some small nutritional differences in organic foods, but they are marginal and won't play a significant difference in overall health. Some organic products have been found to be a bit higher in phosphorus but lower in protein. Organic cow's milk may contain higher levels of omega-3 fatty acids, iron, and vitamin E than nonorganic but, again, less of other nutrients such as selenium and iodine.

Agricultural research is renowned for varying results. The nutrient content of food depends on so many factors, including soil quality, weather conditions, and when the crops are harvested (which differs throughout the world). The composition of

Organic certification

TO MAKE AN ORGANIC CLAIM, A PRODUCT MUST FOLLOW STRICT PRODUCTION, HANDLING, AND LABELING STANDARDS, AND GO THROUGH A CERTIFICATION PROCESS.

The four distinct labeling categories for organic products are: 100 percent organic—made with 100 percent certified organic ingredients; organic—certified organic, except where specified on the National List of Allowed and Prohibited Substance; made with organic ingredients—at least 70 percent of the product is made with certified organic ingredients; and specific organic ingredients—less than 70 percent certified organic content, doesn't need to be certified.

dairy products and meat can also be affected by differences in genetics and what diet animals are fed. Even the natural variations in the production and handling of foods make comparisons difficult. So the results of these studies should be interpreted with caution.

Ultimately, there is not enough strong evidence available to prove that eating organic foods provides added health benefits when compared to eating conventionally farmed foods.

PESTICIDES

Conventional farming relies on the use of chemical pesticides. Although overall they are safe, we are advised to wash our produce before we eat it to remove pesticide residues. Some research suggests that high exposure to pesticides in early life may harm cognitive development, but findings are mixed.

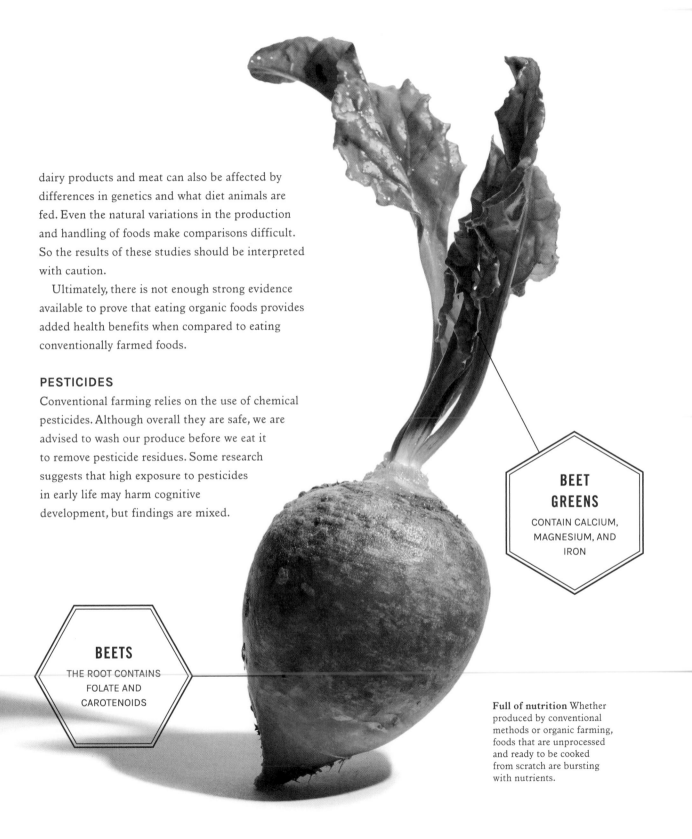

BEET GREENS
CONTAIN CALCIUM, MAGNESIUM, AND IRON

BEETS
THE ROOT CONTAINS FOLATE AND CAROTENOIDS

Full of nutrition Whether produced by conventional methods or organic farming, foods that are unprocessed and ready to be cooked from scratch are bursting with nutrients.

SHOULD I CHANGE MY DIET IF I'M EXERCISING?

Anyone who's getting more serious about fitness can learn from sports nutrition for elite athletes—eat the right balance of food groups for your personal training goals.

Carbohydrate is the main fuel for any exercise; it promotes strength and endurance, delays muscle fatigue, and speeds up recovery, meaning fewer injuries. It is converted to glucose, and excess is stored as glycogen in the liver and muscles, providing instantly available energy. The longer and/or more intense the training, the faster glycogen depletes and fatigue can set in. Resistance training plus protein builds muscle, but without enough carbohydrate, protein will be used for energy instead. Stepping up training can increase appetite, so it's easy to eat more than your body really needs.

FAT

Dietary fat must be converted into fatty acids before being taken up by muscles; it acts as support fuel during low-intensity endurance exercise like long-distance running, when glycogen runs low. Slower availability is also why you should avoid eating fats just before training. At least 15–20 percent of overall calorie intake should come from healthy fats.

PROTEIN

Protein's primary role is to build, and rebuild, muscle. Aim to eat 0.8g–1g per kg/2lb of body weight daily—in the lower range for endurance and higher for strength training. Opt for lean or low-fat foods like skinless chicken and yogurt. Protein is more effectively absorbed from food than supplements.

ENERGY BALANCE

Signs that your diet isn't meeting your energy needs include fatigue, poor sleep quality, and irregular bowel movements.

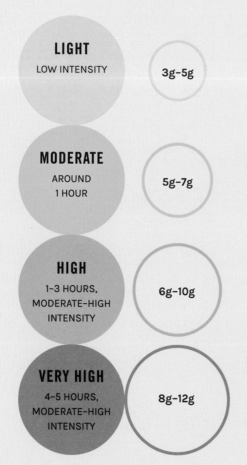

LIGHT
LOW INTENSITY

3g–5g

MODERATE
AROUND
1 HOUR

5g–7g

HIGH
1–3 HOURS,
MODERATE-HIGH
INTENSITY

6g–10g

VERY HIGH
4–5 HOURS,
MODERATE-HIGH
INTENSITY

8g–12g

Daily carbohydrate needs:
This is measured in grams by
1kg (2lb) of body weight, based
on your individual activity level.

HOW IMPORTANT IS HYDRATION?

Proper hydration is essential before, during, and after exercise; otherwise, physical and mental performance can be compromised.

When the body doesn't get enough fluids, the blood thickens, making the heart work less efficiently and increasing heart rate. While some sweat can be lost without affecting your workout, after a point, fluid and sodium loss may impact performance by up to 20 percent. You can feel tired and everything becomes harder.

HYDRATION ZONE

Research shows being properly hydrated when you start training gives the best chance of optimum performance. Drinking 13oz–20oz about two hours beforehand gives the body time to excrete what you don't need and makes up for any previous fluid deficit.

Men should drink around 15.5 cups (3.7 liters) of water daily and women around 11.5 cups (2.7 liters), but you can lose 1.5–4

liters while training. Weigh yourself before and after to see how much you drop through fluid loss, taking into account any fluid consumed during exercise. Aim to stay within 2 percent of your body weight; if you weigh 143lb at the start of your workout, you should weigh no less than 140lb at the end. This is your "hydration zone."

After exercise, for every 2lb (1kg) of water weight lost, gradually drink 5–6 cups of water over about an hour (the extra 1–2 cups compensates for increased urination). A little sodium (salt) in food or drink helps retain fluid.

Drinking too much may cause hyponatraemia, or abnormally low sodium in the blood, which can lead to blackouts and fits. Be aware that symptoms (including lethargy, dizziness, and nausea) can mimic those of dehydration; if these persist, seek medical attention.

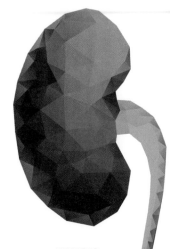

KIDNEYS

Hydration and kidneys: Staying hydrated helps blood deliver nutrients to kidneys and enables them to expel waste as urine.

Hydration and blood

Water in the blood moves between blood cells and blood plasma in a process called osmosis—toward the highest concentration of sodium, in order to equalize their sodium levels.

Sodium   Water   Blood cells

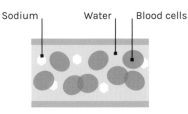
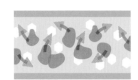
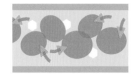

NORMAL SODIUM

When we are well hydrated, sodium levels in both plasma and cells are balanced, ensuring an even pressure between them and supporting normal blood volume and supply.

HYPERNATRAEMIA

If we don't drink enough, sodium levels in plasma rise; in response, water moves from cells into plasma, causing cells to shrink. Symptoms include excessive thirst and fatigue.

HYPONATRAEMIA

If we drink too much too quickly, blood sodium decreases and osmotic pressure moves water from plasma into cells. These swell, leading to "water intoxication."

BLADDER

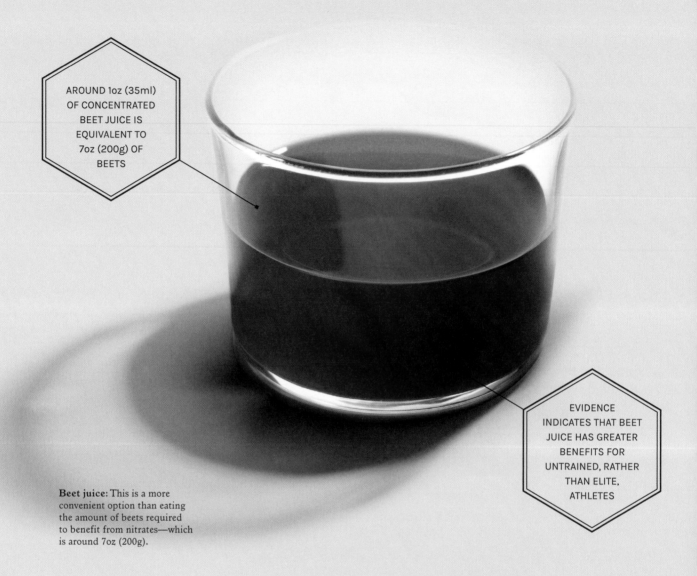

AROUND 1oz (35ml)
OF CONCENTRATED
BEET JUICE IS
EQUIVALENT TO
7oz (200g) OF
BEETS

EVIDENCE
INDICATES THAT BEET
JUICE HAS GREATER
BENEFITS FOR
UNTRAINED, RATHER
THAN ELITE,
ATHLETES

Beet juice: This is a more
convenient option than eating
the amount of beets required
to benefit from nitrates—which
is around 7oz (200g).

DIETARY SOURCES OF LEUCINE (BRANCHED-CHAIN AMINO ACID)

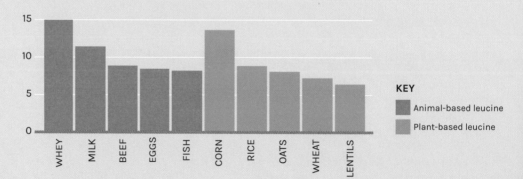

Muscle supporter:
This chart shows leucine
as a percentage of total
protein; you may need to
eat more overall calories
to obtain it from some
foods with lower levels.

KEY

Animal-based leucine

Plant-based leucine

DO I NEED SPORTS SUPPLEMENTS?

If you regularly run or cycle long distances, build muscle strength at the gym, or otherwise train hard, supplementing a healthy, balanced diet can be a good way to fill in nutritional gaps, get extra fuel on workout days, or boost performance.

For most people who visit the gym or play sports recreationally, supplements aren't necessary; they may have a place only if you're on a low-calorie diet or unable to meet your nutritional needs. More intense exercise increases the body's need for certain nutrients, but the International Olympic Committee says even elite athletes should for the most part be able meet their needs by eating a balanced diet. Supplements can be a useful addition to enhance performance, although an excess can potentially cause stomach pain, nausea, and constipation.

BEET JUICE

Beets increase nitrate levels in the blood, which then helps dilate blood vessels and regulate blood pressure so more nutrients and oxygen can reach muscles during exercise, allowing you to sustain higher levels of power for longer. Drink beet juice 2–3 hours before training. Nitrate is also found in veggies like spinach, arugula, broccoli, and cabbage.

BRANCHED-CHAIN AMINO ACIDS (BCAAs)

These are found in protein; leucine and isoleucine support muscle growth and repair and glucose uptake into cells, to fuel body and brain functions. Active people require 0.8g–1g of protein per kg/2lb of body weight per day; there are many food sources of BCAAs, including meat and eggs, although plant sources should be varied (see pages 128–129). The body can use 1g–3g of leucine, or around 20g–40g of protein, per meal for muscle synthesis (from 0.25g to 0.4g of protein per kg/2lb of bodyweight, based on activity levels). While supplements support muscle growth over time, it's cheaper to eat more protein.

PROTEIN POWDER

Only those with high energy requirements need to supplement protein. Whey protein is derived from cow's milk; evidence suggests it's the best form of protein to take after exercise, being absorbed by the body more quickly than others such as casein or soy. (Plant-based supplements combine soy, pea, and rice.) While it's also a good source of leucine, studies show no evidence of greater muscle growth over 24 hours from taking whey protein, as opposed to eating a normal, balanced diet.

CREATINE

Creatine is found in muscle cells, and supplements have proven effectiveness in increasing strength and power, especially for activities involving explosive movements. Red meat, fish, and poultry contain only small amounts of creatine, so supplementing is an option for boosting performance, and for vegetarians and vegans. Of the many types available, creatine monohydrate appears to be an effective option.

WHEN SHOULD I EAT BEFORE EXERCISE?

Just as you wouldn't set off on a long drive very low on fuel, you may need to top off your personal tank before training to get the most from a workout.

Your goal is to have enough stored glycogen from carbohydrates when you start training to sustain performance throughout. If you exercise first thing, glycogen in the liver has been depleted overnight, although some is still present in muscles if your diet contains enough carbohydrates (see pages 78–79). Exercising on a full stomach can be uncomfortable, as blood is directed away from your digestive system.

BEFORE EXERCISING

The consensus is to eat a meal 2–4 hours before working out, where possible. An ideal preworkout meal is mainly carbohydrate with some protein and a little fat, for example, salmon, white rice, and vegetables roasted in olive oil. If you train early and don't have the time or appetite, try a more carb-heavy meal the night before. If you're exercising sooner, or need to top off, a snack (like toast and honey or fruit salad) 1–2 hours beforehand gives a burst of energy for fuel and is quickly absorbed. With under an hour, stick to liquids like smoothies or sports drinks. Experiment to find the optimal timing for your activity, schedule, and digestion.

DURING EXERCISE

Water should suffice for 45–75-minute sessions. After an hour, you may want to consume around 30g of carbs per hour for two hours, increasing to 60g per hour for the next 2–2.5 hours. Gels and sports drinks can help maintain blood sugar levels but can also contribute to stomach upset during endurance activities like distance running; practice what works for you.

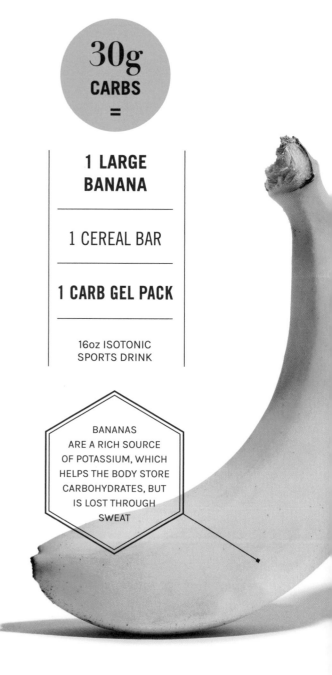

30g CARBS =

1 LARGE BANANA

1 CEREAL BAR

1 CARB GEL PACK

16oz ISOTONIC SPORTS DRINK

BANANAS ARE A RICH SOURCE OF POTASSIUM, WHICH HELPS THE BODY STORE CARBOHYDRATES, BUT IS LOST THROUGH SWEAT

IS IT BETTER TO REFUEL RIGHT AFTER EXERCISE?

The more frequently and intensively you train, the more important it is to replenish fluid and fuel afterward to avoid aching muscles, fatigue, and underperformance.

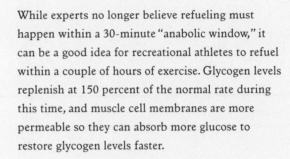

POST WORKOUT

FOR CARBS AND PROTEIN, A FRUIT SMOOTHIE WITH OATS, YOGURT, AND MILK IS IDEAL

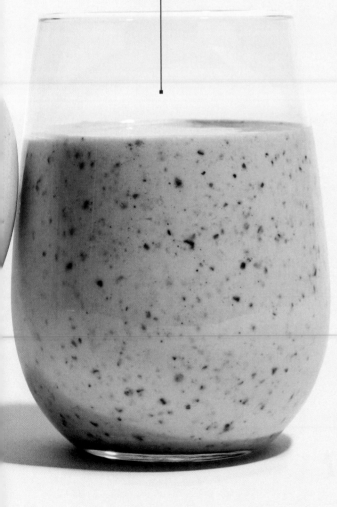

While experts no longer believe refueling must happen within a 30-minute "anabolic window," it can be a good idea for recreational athletes to refuel within a couple of hours of exercise. Glycogen levels replenish at 150 percent of the normal rate during this time, and muscle cell membranes are more permeable so they can absorb more glucose to restore glycogen levels faster.

CARB–PROTEIN BALANCE

Recovery foods should contain quality carbohydrates to replenish glycogen and fluid and electrolytes to rehydrate effectively. In addition, combining a small amount of protein with carbs postworkout has been shown to more effectively promote glycogen recovery than carbohydrates alone. Flavored milks, smoothies, and fruit yogurts all check these boxes. Choose the fat and sugar content based on your individual body composition and energy needs.

If your training is mainly strength based, or if you're training at a high intensity, there is evidence that adding 15g–25g of protein to a postworkout meal or snack can reduce muscle soreness and promote muscle repair. (A 150g serving of edamame would provide this.)

Otherwise, follow your food preferences, appetite, and what sits comfortably in your stomach after exercise, and eat when you feel hungry. Overall daily energy and macronutrient intake is the priority; provided you consume enough calories, carbs, and protein over a 24-hour period, your muscles should recover before exercising again (see pages 78–79).

WILL I LOSE WEIGHT FASTER IF I EXERCISE?

Rapid weight loss is a popular goal, although generally the faster this happens, the less sustainable it is. If you're already restricting calories, is exercise the missing piece in the puzzle of how to successfully reduce weight long term?

Exercise burns extra calories, and expending more energy than we consume creates an energy deficit that leads to weight loss. In practice, though, exercising doesn't guarantee less body fat. One reason may be unrealistic expectations; a study found people overestimated calories burned during exercise by 2–3 times the actual amount.

EXERCISE AND METABOLISM

Several investigations have shown huge variations in individual responses to exercise—this is because its effect on appetite depends on your hormones, body fat levels, and metabolism. The largest proportion of energy intake is used for basic physiological functions while doing nothing—your resting metabolic rate (RMR). Physical activity, including exercise, uses 10–30 percent, so its impact is limited.

Rapid weight loss can cause loss of muscle and slow your metabolic rate (see pages 92–93). Doing

some weight-based exercise to build muscle may help offset this because muscle uses more energy—if you don't consume extra calories. Sleep quality and stress also play a role in appetite and activity levels.

CAN I JUST EXERCISE?

Studies indicate that while aerobic (cardio) exercise burns fat, diet has a bigger impact on weight loss than exercise. Combining exercise with diet appears to be more effective over both the short and long term. However, exercise is beneficial for maintaining lower weight; people who have done so for five years report exercising daily.

What's not in doubt are the many long-term health benefits of regular exercise. These include significantly reduced risk of heart disease, stroke, colon cancer, depression, and early death.

One study defines successful weight loss as losing at least 10 percent of initial body weight

Energy balance equation
Weight loss requires a negative energy balance, with fewer calories eaten than used by resting metabolic rate, exercise, other non-exercise activity (NEAT), and the thermic effect of food (TEF), or energy used to digest it.

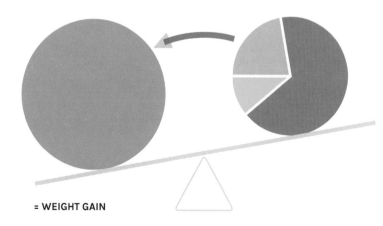

= WEIGHT GAIN

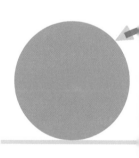

NEUTRAL (WEIGHT MANAGEMENT)

Calculate your calorie needs

To get a rough idea of your body's daily energy needs, first figure out your resting metabolic rate, then multiply by the appropriate activity factor.

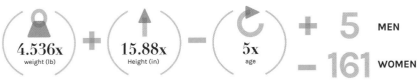

Example: Male 165lb, 72in, age 40, moderately active:
(4.536 x 165) + (15.88 x 72) − (5 x 40) + 5 = 1,697kcals
1,697kcals x 1.55 = **2,630 calories**

* Based on the Harris-Benedict equation

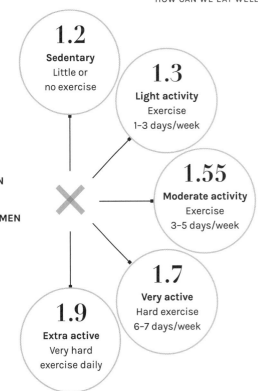

and keeping it off for one year. This suggests the best approach is slowly increasing the amount and intensity of exercise so it becomes an enjoyable lifestyle habit and your body has time to adapt.

ACTIVE LIVING

Non-exercise activity thermogenesis (NEAT) is the energy expended when we aren't sleeping, eating, or exercising. Small daily changes in behavior, like standing up while reading or taking stairs, can all boost NEAT. One research review even estimated higher-level NEAT activities (like washing windows) could burn up to 2,000 calories extra daily. But fatigue resulting from exercise can also reduce NEAT.

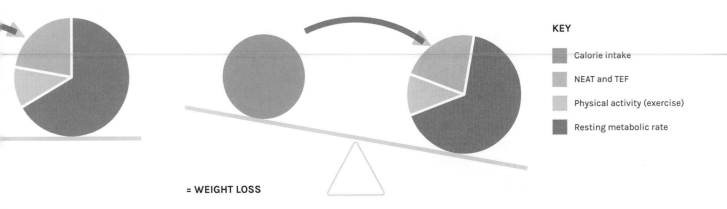

KEY

- Calorie intake
- NEAT and TEF
- Physical activity (exercise)
- Resting metabolic rate

= WEIGHT LOSS

WHICH EXERCISE IS BETTER AT FAT BURNING?

Body fat is distributed within muscles, around organs, and beneath skin, which means you can't target specific areas of the body. However, you may have heard that some types of exercise are better for burning fat—do such shortcuts really exist?

When working out at lower intensities, like walking or steady running, your body will predominantly burn fat for fuel. In the gym, the "fat-burning" zone is usually indicated on a heart rate chart on cardio equipment like rowing machines and stair climbers. Staying within this zone keeps your heart rate, and your intensity, relatively low. This burns more calories from stored body fat rather than glycogen in the muscles and liver, and glucose in blood (both derived from carbohydrates). However, you'll burn more calories overall—and therefore lose more weight—by working at a higher intensity for as long and as often as you can safely manage (supported by diet so you're in an energy deficit; see pages 84–85).

FASTED CARDIO

Cardio exercise, like cycling, power-walking, running, and aerobics, raises your heart rate. Some studies have shown doing cardio on an empty stomach increases the rate of fat burning, because glycogen stores are depleted so the body takes more energy from fat. However, this may also cause breakdown of muscle tissue and increased appetite.

INTERVAL TRAINING

Combining bursts of high-intensity exercise like sprinting with intervals of less intense activity is often promoted as more effective for fat burning than maintaining a continuous moderate intensity,

Target heart rate

To ensure you're working at your target intensity, place your index and middle fingers on your pulse, count for 30 seconds, and multiply by two for your heart rate in BPM (beats per minute).

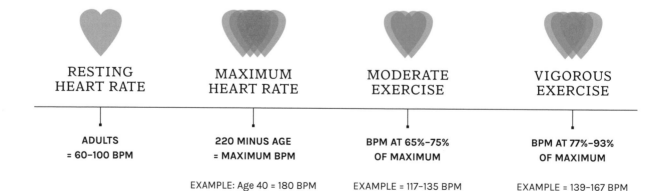

RESTING HEART RATE	MAXIMUM HEART RATE	MODERATE EXERCISE	VIGOROUS EXERCISE
ADULTS = 60-100 BPM	220 MINUS AGE = MAXIMUM BPM	BPM AT 65%–75% OF MAXIMUM	BPM AT 77%–93% OF MAXIMUM
	EXAMPLE: Age 40 = 180 BPM	EXAMPLE = 117-135 BPM	EXAMPLE = 139-167 BPM

for instance, by jogging. However, a 2017 analysis of 31 studies found high-intensity interval training resulted in similar body fat reduction as continuous moderate-intensity training—and maintaining a moderate pace for longer was more beneficial than shorter periods of interval training.

Overall, evidence suggests interval training is better for improving overall fitness and respiratory and cardiovascular health than burning fat—unless you can sustain it for long enough.

SWITCH INTENSITIES

It's sensible to mix up different intensities in your workout, to keep it interesting and to avoid injury. While weight-based resistance training is used to build muscle rather than burn fat, having more muscle can promote better fat burning when you're not exercising (see pages 84–85).

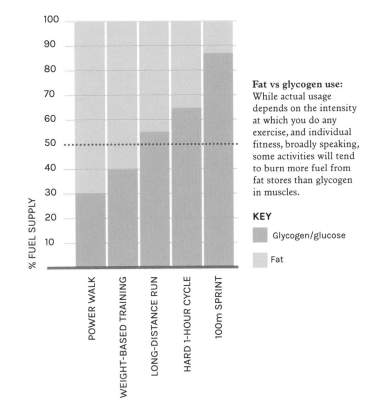

Fat vs glycogen use: While actual usage depends on the intensity at which you do any exercise, and individual fitness, broadly speaking, some activities will tend to burn more fuel from fat stores than glycogen in muscles.

KEY

▨ Glycogen/glucose

▨ Fat

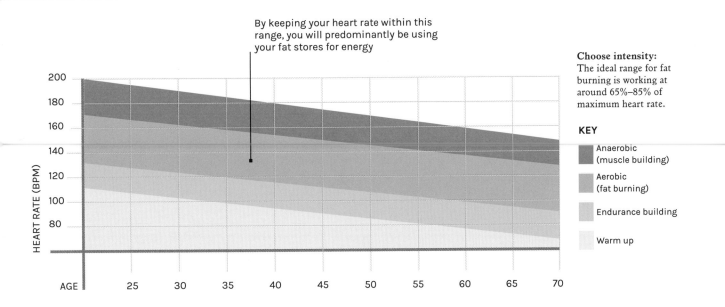

By keeping your heart rate within this range, you will predominantly be using your fat stores for energy

Choose intensity: The ideal range for fat burning is working at around 65%–85% of maximum heart rate.

KEY

■ Anaerobic (muscle building)

■ Aerobic (fat burning)

■ Endurance building

■ Warm up

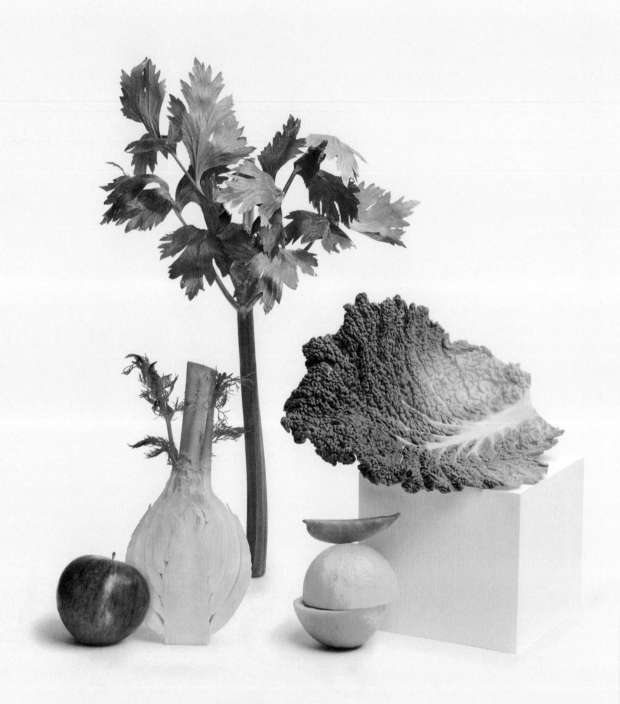

SHOULD I GO ON A DIET?

IS IT GOOD TO BE SLIM?

"Slim" is just one of many cultural constructs about how our bodies should look. But achieving these ideals and being a healthy weight aren't necessarily related.

Body size and shape aren't always the best indicator of health. Someone who eats a less healthy diet and does little exercise may be genetically predetermined to have less body fat than someone in a larger body leading a healthier lifestyle. Scientists have identified specific DNA variants common to people with obesity, and in 2019 researchers found that obese people have a higher genetic risk score than those at a "normal" weight.

A large body of evidence indicates that you are less likely to experience poor long-term health if you don't carry too much fat relative to your height and build. For example, being overweight makes you three times more likely to develop type 2 diabetes (seven times for those with obesity), while people who are overweight in middle age have a 35 percent increased risk of Alzheimer's disease. Obesity is a risk factor for poor sleep, joint and bone problems, chronic noncommunicable diseases like cancer and coronary heart disease, and mental health disorders. In contrast, healthy weight individuals have improved fertility and greater chances of conceiving (see page 182).

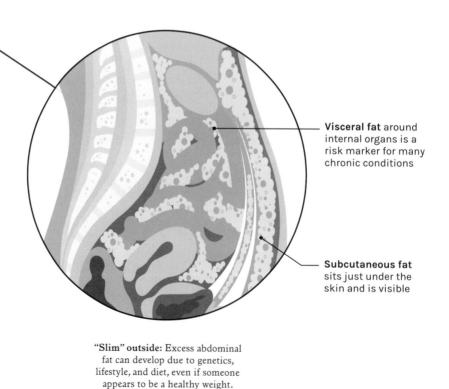

Visceral fat around internal organs is a risk marker for many chronic conditions

Subcutaneous fat sits just under the skin and is visible

"Slim" outside: Excess abdominal fat can develop due to genetics, lifestyle, and diet, even if someone appears to be a healthy weight.

Measuring BMI

BMI expresses weight relative to height; however, very fit people like professional football players can have BMIs that appear unhealthy due to a high muscle-to-fat ratio. To calculate BMI, divide weight in pounds by height in square inches and multiply by 703: 212lb / (72.8in x 72.8in) x 703 = 28.

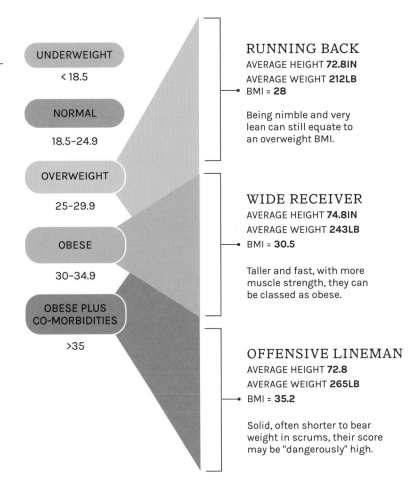

UNDERWEIGHT

< 18.5

NORMAL

18.5–24.9

OVERWEIGHT

25–29.9

OBESE

30–34.9

OBESE PLUS CO-MORBIDITIES

>35

RUNNING BACK
AVERAGE HEIGHT **72.8IN**
AVERAGE WEIGHT **212LB**
BMI = **28**

Being nimble and very lean can still equate to an overweight BMI.

WIDE RECEIVER
AVERAGE HEIGHT **74.8IN**
AVERAGE WEIGHT **243LB**
BMI = **30.5**

Taller and fast, with more muscle strength, they can be classed as obese.

OFFENSIVE LINEMAN
AVERAGE HEIGHT **72.8**
AVERAGE WEIGHT **265LB**
BMI = **35.2**

Solid, often shorter to bear weight in scrums, their score may be "dangerously" high.

"HEALTHY" WEIGHT

There are different measures of "healthy" and "overweight." BMI (body mass index) is widely used by health professionals and has a strong correlation with various diseases and chronic conditions. However, it doesn't reflect the amount of fat or muscle in a body, bone weight, or cultural factors, age, and gender (women tend to carry more fat). Waist circumference is another commonly used measure because excess abdominal fat—more than 40 inches for men and 35 inches for women—increases the risk of developing obesity-related conditions. While both are used to screen for potential risk, they aren't diagnostic tools.

Instead of using weight or measures like BMI to define well-being, an alternative "health at every size" approach focuses on sustainable health-promoting behavior regardless of body size. Proponents argue a weight-neutral approach is healthier because it avoids the potentially harmful effects of repeated dieting, such as a higher risk of early death and psychological distress. Ultimately, nutrition and health are socioeconomic issues that require understanding and empathy.

IS THERE A LIMIT TO HOW MUCH WEIGHT I CAN LOSE?

Numerous studies have observed that when some people try to lose weight, their body appears to hold onto fat and may not let them either reach a target weight or sustain it long term. As yet, scientists don't know precisely why this happens.

For many people, trying to lose weight works initially, then they hit a plateau and stop, or they reach their target weight only to find it rises again and they end up gaining pounds. Analysis of 29 long-term weight-loss studies found that more than half of lost weight was regained within two years, and over 80 percent within five.

SET POINT

Set point theory says this happens because we have a narrow, genetically determined range of weight the body is programmed to protect. When the brain detects fat levels have fallen below an established level, it adjusts certain hormones in order to burn energy more slowly and increase calorie intake. (These include leptin, a hormone in fat cells that helps suppress appetite, and ghrelin, which stimulates it.) As weight is regained, the weight range is set higher to protect fat stores. Scientists think these compensating mechanisms may keep working for up to a year. Some research also suggests repeated dieting means we develop resistance to key hormones, making it even harder to lose weight.

The set point concept is supported by significant observational study. But it doesn't explain the relatively fast increase in Western populations' body weight and adiposity (excess fat) since the 1980s, or why obesity levels vary with socioeconomic status.

SETTLING POINT

This newer theory says body weight gradually settles at a level reflecting our genetics but also any significant changes in our diet, activity, environment, lifestyle, and stress levels. There is research supporting both theories; taken together, they suggest that we have a predetermined weight range, but other factors can influence and change it.

CAN I RESET?

Based on current evidence, weight loss can be maintained, but a gradual process is more effective. Losing a pound or two a week allows your body to adapt and is sustainable in the long run. This means eating fewer calories than you use but in a way that's realistic, for example, by adding more vegetables to your diet and walking more rather than spending hours in the gym every day. Studies show increased physical activity positively affects body composition, but weight loss is individual and your body may react differently from someone else's.

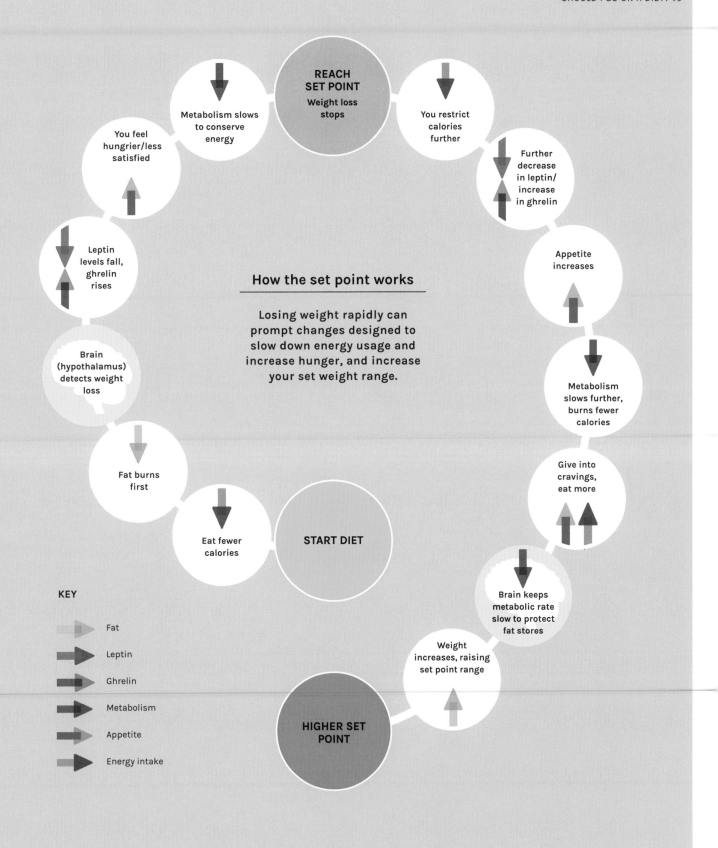

REACH
SET POINT
Weight loss
stops

Metabolism slows
to conserve
energy

You feel
hungrier/less
satisfied

You restrict
calories
further

Further
decrease
in leptin/
increase
in ghrelin

Leptin
levels fall,
ghrelin
rises

Appetite
increases

How the set point works

Losing weight rapidly can
prompt changes designed to
slow down energy usage and
increase hunger, and increase
your set weight range.

Brain
(hypothalamus)
detects weight
loss

Metabolism
slows further,
burns fewer
calories

Fat burns
first

Give into
cravings,
eat more

Eat fewer
calories

START DIET

Brain keeps
metabolic rate
slow to protect
fat stores

Weight
increases, raising
set point range

KEY

Fat

Leptin

Ghrelin

Metabolism

Appetite

Energy intake

HIGHER SET
POINT

IF DIETS DON'T WORK, WHAT DOES?

"Dieting" is often unsustainable, with one analysis of 14 popular diet programs finding that weight loss was mostly reversed after 12 months. By understanding how the concept affects our thinking, we can identify more effective approaches.

As babies, we are in tune with our body's hunger signals and eat only what we need, but as we age, we're surrounded by messaging and social pressures around food and lose this innate ability. The complex psychology surrounding our relationship with food undoubtedly plays a role in the failure of diets and can be the biggest barrier to weight loss.

Research shows that restrained eaters experience more intense food cravings, heightened emotions surrounding food, and greater preoccupation with it. Likewise, categorizing foods as "good" or "bad" creates a restrictive mindset that increases food cravings and, in turn, the risk of overeating these foods when they are available. Labeling foods as treats implies they can be eaten only once earned, which increases desire. Goal setting can also have detrimental psychological effects, as veering "off plan" can prompt feelings of failure and guilt and subsequent overeating.

SLOW AND STEADY

Studies show that slow, steady weight loss over a longer time period is the most effective way to lose body fat. According to one study, sustained adherence to a diet—rather than following a certain type of diet—is the key to successful weight management. Instead of cutting out entire meals and risking fatigue and cravings, aim to control your portion sizes at each meal and choose healthier snacks between meals. Eating more variety is also thought to enhance weight loss; try different types of meals and vegetables each day.

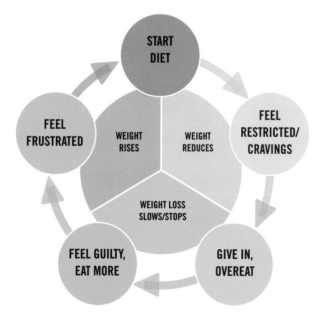

The psychological diet cycle
Dieting can set up a mindset of succeeding or failing, which may then lead to potentially harmful yo-yo dieting.

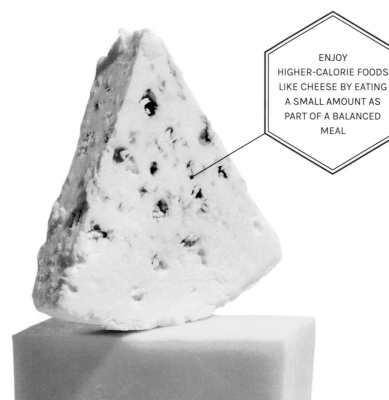

ENJOY HIGHER-CALORIE FOODS LIKE CHEESE BY EATING A SMALL AMOUNT AS PART OF A BALANCED MEAL

ALONGSIDE FAT, A THUMB-SIZE PIECE OF HARD CHEESE PROVIDES AROUND 180mg OF CALCIUM AND 8g OF PROTEIN

GOAT CHEESE, BRIE, AND CAMEMBERT SHOULD BE EATEN LESS OFTEN THAN LOWER FAT AND SALT OPTIONS LIKE RICOTTA AND COTTAGE CHEESE

WHAT WORKS

- Eat a healthy, balanced diet (see pages 40–41).
- Practice portion control.
- Eat less-healthy foods that you enjoy only occasionally.
- Listen to your body—eat when you're hungry and stop when you're full.
- Exercise regularly, ideally 30 minutes daily.
- Try some strategies to manage stress; it increases the hormone cortisol, which lowers blood sugar and increases food cravings.
- Get enough sleep; this will help control cortisol.

"Bad" food: Cheese is often ruled out when trying to lose weight, but its fat content can help you feel satisfied and it contains protein, vitamins, and minerals.

HOW DO I FIND A WEIGHT-LOSS PROGRAM THAT WORKS FOR ME?

Rather than following a formal diet plan, fixating on calories, or avoiding particular foods, reaching and maintaining a healthy weight means finding a way of eating that works for your needs—maybe with some professional help.

Although there are many weight-loss plans to choose from, we don't all respond to one-size-fits-all diets in the same way. A 2020 study into the three main types of programs (low carbohydrate, high protein, and low fat) concluded that none is more effective and results varied with each individual. Other research has demonstrated that the quality of the food we eat is an important factor in achieving and maintaining a healthy weight. "A calorie is a calorie" doesn't tell the whole story; we need to consider each food's overall nutritional facts and our habits over time.

PERSONALIZING NUTRITION

Studies on individualized nutrition are rare, but scientists conducting a large-scale and long-term observational study called Project 10K are looking at how participants respond to different foods, the makeup of their gut bacteria, and whether they should eat to suit their DNA. Results may lead to more research supporting personalized nutrition and eating for better health outcomes.

Meanwhile, the ideal nutritional plan should provide flexibility and room for socializing, address emotional and physical needs, and help you feel good. It will consider:

- What "healthy" means to you—maybe eating more greens or just less sugar
- How active you are and how often you exercise
- Your food preferences, knowledge, and concerns
- Your physical and mental health, including sleep quality, hormone function, and anxiety levels
- Your social, cultural, and family influences
- Realistic goals and support

Keep a food diary

This is a good way to learn more about your personal eating patterns. It will help you understand how different people, times, events, and your mood, affect your intake.

WHICH FOOD

Be specific
List each intake in detail, for example, "Cup of coffee: 1 tsp sugar, 2tsp fat-free milk."

HOW FILLING

Full and satisfied?
Score/10 your enjoyment and how hungry you felt before and after eating.

WHAT TIME

Timing triggers
Was it a planned meal, a regular snack, or an impulse?

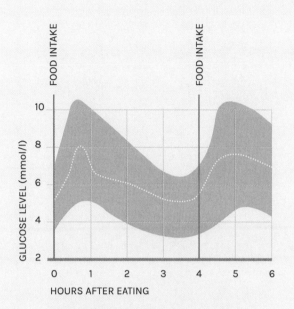

EFFECT OF FOOD ON DIFFERENT PEOPLE'S
BLOOD GLUCOSE

Varying responses to food:
A study of more than 1,000
people found eating the same
meal caused a much bigger
blood sugar spike for some,
showing the ideal nutritional
plan should take individual
biology into account to be
sustainable long term.

KEY

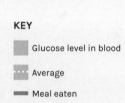

Glucose level in blood

Average

Meal eaten

PROFESSIONAL ADVICE

Registered dietitian nutritionists and qualified
nutritionists can provide guidance on losing weight
sustainably, as well as helping with other health and
fitness issues. You'll be questioned in depth about
your health and history with food and what your
goals are, and you may be asked to keep a food or
lifestyle journal. Write down any questions you have
beforehand, as it can be overwhelming discussing
your life and eating habits at first. You should leave
your session with notes, advice on next steps, and,
in most cases, a scheduled follow-up appointment.

Professional advice can be expensive; alternative
options include self- and group-help programs and
online planning tools.

WHERE

Location eating
We often eat
habitually in
certain places.

WHO WAS THERE

Being polite?
Over-/undereating can be
linked to certain people,
events, or social customs.

WHAT YOU WERE DOING

Food or fuel?
Are you refueling at the
gym or busy at work?

HOW YOU FEEL

Food and mood
Note how you were feeling
before consuming and if it
affected your mood.

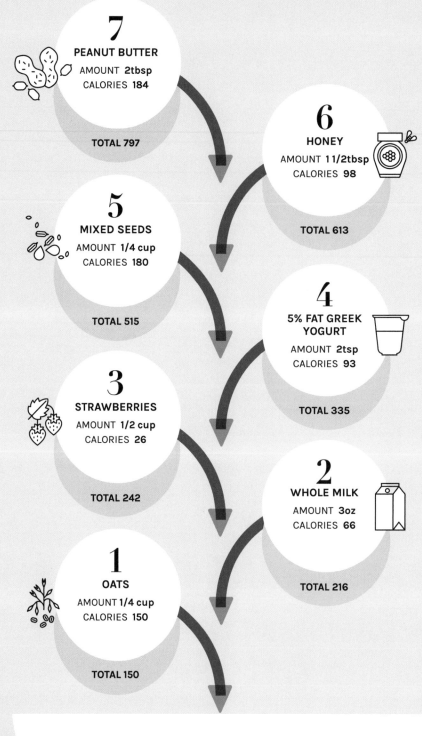

7
PEANUT BUTTER
AMOUNT **2tbsp**
CALORIES **184**
TOTAL 797

6
HONEY
AMOUNT **1 1/2tbsp**
CALORIES **98**
TOTAL 613

5
MIXED SEEDS
AMOUNT **1/4 cup**
CALORIES **180**
TOTAL 515

4
5% FAT GREEK YOGURT
AMOUNT **2tsp**
CALORIES **93**
TOTAL 335

3
STRAWBERRIES
AMOUNT **1/2 cup**
CALORIES **26**
TOTAL 242

2
WHOLE MILK
AMOUNT **3oz**
CALORIES **66**
TOTAL 216

1
OATS
AMOUNT **1/4 cup**
CALORIES **150**
TOTAL 150

Build a bowl

By adding relatively small amounts of nutrient-dense foods to a meal, in this case breakfast, you can boost your calorie intake without having to eat too much.

DO I NEED TO GAIN WEIGHT?

Labels like "too thin" and "skinny" can be just as toxic as those put onto heavier people, especially if you are naturally in a smaller body. However, adding fat or muscle to your body is not as simple as increasing portion sizes.

Gaining weight is a complex issue. BMI (body mass index) is a standard measure for whether someone is overweight, healthy weight, or—if the score is less than 18.5—underweight. However, a 2019 study of 2,000 subjects with BMIs under 18 found that 75 percent of them were genetically predisposed to be underweight and were examples of "healthy thinness." So you may have no need to gain weight, even if your BMI indicates you should. (Although someone with a low BMI who appears healthy may still need to put on weight for optimal health.)

THE ROLE OF GENETICS

Some people are naturally underweight or smaller because their bodies are not set up to store adipose tissue, where lipids (fats) accumulate. Genes also play a role in our ability to grow muscles, which then affects how rapidly we burn energy. It's often said that people in smaller bodies have great metabolisms; in fact, the larger and more muscular you are, the harder your metabolism works and the more calories you burn. Smaller people's capacity for gaining weight partially depends upon their muscle mass. If this is high, they can find it more difficult to put on weight.

HEALTH IMPACT

Genetics aside, you may be under a healthy weight for your body for other reasons, such as stress, illness, or an eating disorder (see pages 32–33).

Weighing too little can lead to fatigue and health problems like a weakened immune system, fragile bones, and missed periods. This may be because you are not eating enough to get enough key nutrients, such as calcium. Some people may not even be aware they are under their optimal body weight; warning signs that you may be include:

● Suppressed appetite
● Irregular bathroom habits, especially going less
● Thinning hair, hair loss, or dry skin
● Regularly feeling unwell

GAIN WEIGHT SAFELY

Simply eating more won't work; the types of food you eat and your activity levels also need to adjust. Talk to your doctor or a registered dietitian about gaining weight safely and sustainably. Broadly speaking, aim for 1–2lb of weight gain a week and do some low-intensity exercise. Eating more to gain weight can be challenging; to reduce portions, add some nutrient-dense foods that are high in calories, fat, or sugar, into a balanced diet, such as:

● Starchy (ideally whole grain) carbs like potatoes, bread, pasta, and rice
● Full-fat milk (until your weight begins to rise)
● Unsaturated oils and spreads
● Nuts, seeds, and avocados for healthy fats
● Beans, eggs, pulses, meat, and fish for protein
● Yogurts, homemade milkshakes, and puddings for protein and calories.

SHOULD I COUNT CALORIES?

Counting helps build awareness of our daily energy consumption. But food is more than calories, and reducing it to a number risks oversimplifying its nourishment.

———————

Monitoring calories can help you reach the energy deficit needed to lose weight. However, not all calories are nutritionally equal. Also, the body metabolizes foods differently; for instance, it may absorb more calories from a corn tortilla than from an equivalent amount of sweet corn (some of which may be visible in your toilet the next day!). In addition, calories may be more available to one person than to another.

UNHEALTHY COUNTING

As well as being time consuming, calorie counting can lead to restrictive behaviors or unhealthy habits. It may be tempting to eat highly processed foods because calories are clearly displayed on packaging and easier to count, or to exclude nutrient-dense foods like oily fish and nuts purely on the basis of their calorie content.

TRACKING TOOLS

Many people count using a fitness tracker; while these encourage regular activity, one study found that popular brands can overestimate the number of calories burned while walking by more than 50 percent. Relying strictly on these tools, rather than using them to broadly gauge your energy intake and expenditure, could result in overconsumption. Some apps are designed for continuous engagement, which may encourage compulsive logging. If you choose to count, do it within a healthy, balanced diet and listen to your body's hunger cues.

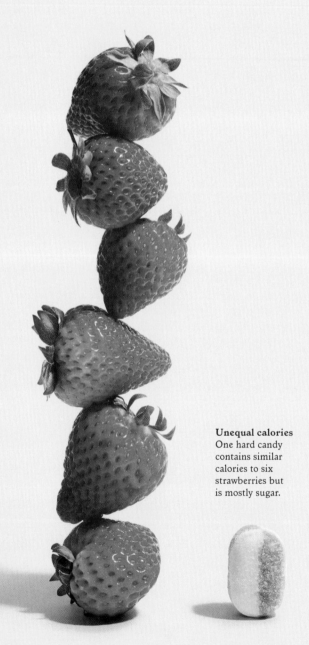

Unequal calories
One hard candy contains similar calories to six strawberries but is mostly sugar.

CAN I RELY ON THE SCALE?

If you're trying to lose weight, stepping onto the scale feels
like a moment of truth. But the number doesn't show what's actually
happening in your body.

Weighing yourself is a simple way to monitor your behavior and make small adjustments to improve your energy balance (see pages 84–85). A research review indicated that daily weighing is associated with more weight loss than less frequent weighing. However, there are a number of reasons it's best not to rely on the scale for measuring weight loss.

WEIGHT VARIABLES

Your weight can fluctuate after just one meal, and 2–6lb over a day. We're often heavier in the evening after eating and drinking; salt, alcohol, medication, and menstruation can also cause water retention. One study found that weight is highest after the weekend and the ideal weigh-in time is Wednesday morning before consuming anything. If you want to establish a rough base weight, use the same scale, at the same time, without clothes.

In addition, overreliance on the scale could contribute to an unhealthy body image and relationship with food, and for some people it can become a crutch.

WHAT DOESN'T THE SCALE TELL ME?

Be mindful that a weight reading doesn't reflect how much body fat you are carrying, your overall body composition, or how healthy you are. Even if the number on the scale isn't falling, you could still be losing body fat, gaining muscle, sleeping better, and improving your gut health (see pages 48–51).

So-called smart scales claim to measure body fat by sending a tiny electrical current through the body. Unfortunately, it's not that simple; for example, if you are dehydrated, these can overestimate the amount of body fat. Most research conducted has concluded that they aren't accurate.

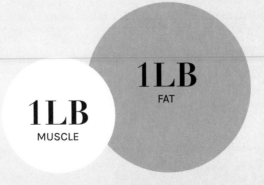

1LB FAT

1LB MUSCLE

Fat vs muscle
Muscle is more dense and takes up less space than fat; with more muscle, you weigh more but look leaner.

ARE MEALTIMES IMPORTANT?

Whether it's making time for breakfast in the morning or sitting down with family to eat dinner in the evening, research suggests that when and how we eat affects both our mental and physical health.

OPTION 1

REGULAR MEAL AT BREAKFAST

REGULAR MEAL AT LUNCH

SMALL MEAL AT DINNER

OPTION 2

SMALL MEAL AT BREAKFAST

REGULAR MEAL AT LUNCH

SMALL MEAL AT DINNER

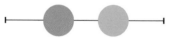

OPTION 3

REGULAR MEAL IN MORNING

REGULAR MEAL IN AFTERNOON

A number of studies have shown that it is healthier to eat meals at the same time each day. Evidence suggests that a regular meal pattern that includes eating breakfast, having 2–3 meals a day, and consuming a greater proportion of your daily energy intake earlier on in the day may have physiological benefits such as reduced inflammation and improved stress resistance. Regular mealtimes provide a sense of rhythm and familiarity, which can have real psychological benefits.

Breakfast

A RECENT STUDY LOOKING AT IRREGULAR BREAKFAST EATING FOUND THAT THOSE AGED BETWEEN 13–18 YEARS WERE THE MOST LIKELY TO SKIP BREAKFAST, with 22 percent of participants in this age group consuming breakfast on 2 days or fewer out of 4. Previous studies have suggested that differences in family structure, ethnicity, socioeconomic status, time constraints, and lack of food enjoyment can all influence this.

Appetite and energy expenditure follow the circadian rhythm, the natural "body clock" that regulates when we wake, sleep, and many things in between. At the same time, the timing of your meals may have an effect on your circadian rhythm. Personalizing your mealtimes to align with your sleep cycle can improve health and limit weight gain.

MAKING THE MOST OF MEALTIMES

Aim to eat sitting at a table and upright in a chair. This position allows your stomach to empty, helping digestion. It also encourages us to eat more mindfully (see pages 206–207) and notice feelings of satiety and fullness (see page 104). Even better is sitting down to eat with friends or family for some social interaction. Having a conversation during a meal slows down the speed at which you eat, meaning you are more likely to notice feelings of fullness before overeating. Conversely, eating dinner in front of the television not only eliminates the opportunity for social interaction but also distracts us from what we are eating, with research suggesting this can cause us to eat more than we need.

IS SNACKING BAD FOR YOU?

Snacking is an often-vilified habit, but it can be practiced
in a way that helps, rather than hinders, good nutrition.

It is extremely common to snack between meals, with reports finding that 94 percent of people in the US and 66 percent in the UK do so at least once a day. Snacking is not in itself bad for you; it can help maintain energy levels, especially during busy days, and prevent you from feeling so hungry that you overeat.

However, snacking can become a habit and even start to replace meals, which is never a good thing, since your body cannot get all the nutrients you need just from small snacks. Many people snack due to boredom, a form of hedonic hunger (see page 104). Eating simply for pleasure is not necessarily a bad thing; after all, food is more than just fuel. But if you choose foods such as cookies, sweets, and cake, which are high in sugar and fat, or snack frequently throughout the day, you may be consuming more than your body needs. On top of this, the snack-food industry often uses disingenuous marketing. While individually wrapped snack bars may be convenient, especially when you are on the go, many of these contain high quantities of sugar, despite being marketed as a "healthy" option (see pages 62–63).

There is no need to avoid certain foods altogether when it comes to snacks, but the best policy is "everything in moderation." Snacking mindfully (see pages 206–207) and choosing healthy, balanced options is a good idea, as this will prevent blood sugar spikes (see pages 202–203) and keep you fuller for longer.

A modern trend

ONE REPORT FOUND THAT MILLENNIALS (THOSE AGED 21–38) ARE MORE LIKELY TO SNACK THAN OLDER GENERATIONS.
Almost a quarter of this age group were found to snack at least four times a day, with a significant proportion of those questioned snacking to deal with boredom or stress.

HEALTHY SNACKS:

- Carrot sticks and hummus
- Chopped apple with 1 tsp of peanut butter
- Small handful of nuts
- A banana and yogurt
- Homemade energy balls
- Rice cakes with avocado

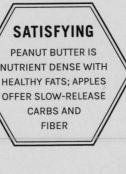

SATISFYING
PEANUT BUTTER IS NUTRIENT DENSE WITH HEALTHY FATS; APPLES OFFER SLOW-RELEASE CARBS AND FIBER

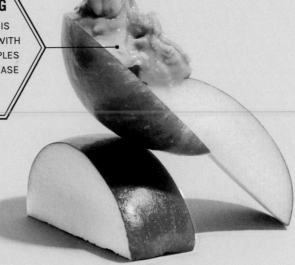

WHY DO I FEEL HUNGRY ALL THE TIME?

It may be because of the simple reason that you need to eat more food! Or perhaps you are misinterpreting your body's signals. Hunger is a much-misunderstood phenomenon.

We've all experienced hunger—the sensation your body produces when you are in need of fuel and nourishment. Satiety refers to feeling full, while satiation refers to feeling satisfied.

Hormones control the balance between hunger and satiety, and what you eat affects the balance of those hormones. Food makes changes to levels of gut hormones, which in turn impacts the metabolites in the blood and the signals they transmit in the body.

TYPES OF HUNGER

Homeostatic hunger refers to the physical feeling of wanting to eat, caused by the need for energy (see opposite). Hedonic hunger describes the desire to eat for pleasure. When we smell or eat something tasty, the brain releases pleasure hormones like dopamine. We then associate that food with the feeling of pleasure we experienced, making us want to eat it again, or eat more of it than we need.

Psychological and emotional factors affect the balance between hunger hormones in ways we don't yet fully understand. Tiredness can also have an impact (see pages 142–143). The human body has a complex system of hormones that interact in myriad ways. For example, cortisol, a stress hormone, suppresses appetite, but in cases of chronic stress, it can enhance appetite.

MANAGING PERSISTENT HUNGER

It seems as we age, we lose connection with our innate hunger signals. For instance, people easily confuse thirst for hunger. Fighting against feeling hungry can do more harm than good, but it's good to recognize and acknowledge whether your body is actually in need of fuel or if your hunger is actually for the pleasure you associate with food.

If you feel tired and your stomach is growling, it's likely your body lacks energy and you need to refuel to satiety. If this happens often, eat a little more at mealtimes, consider increasing your carbohydrate intake, or take a snack with you when out and about.

If it's hedonic hunger that you keep feeling, it's likely you're in need of satiation. Research suggest some types of food can be more satiating than others. A diet rich in fiber or high in protein suppresses ghrelin (the hunger hormone) effectively.

AVOID "I'VE BLOWN IT!" MENTALITY

A destructive pattern emerges with excessive hunger when you give up fighting it and continue to eat beyond the point of fullness, out of a tangled blend of conflicting feelings like desire, guilt, frustration, and fulfillment. If you are struggling to detect your internal cues, try mindful eating and intuitive eating (see pages 208–211). Minimize distractions while eating. For example, turn off the TV.

A satiating square of chocolate after dinner is fine, but if you find yourself overeating or eating out of boredom, step back and take a moment to listen to your body and consider whether you are actually hungry. Often the craving will pass. Distract yourself from the feeling with a different activity.

Chewing food for longer may help you eat less during the meal and feel more satiated afterward.

Hunger hormones

Appetite is governed by the balance of several hormones, notably ghrelin and leptin. Receptors for these in the hypothalamus in the brain respond to their presence by setting off bodily processes that cause sensations of hunger or satiety.

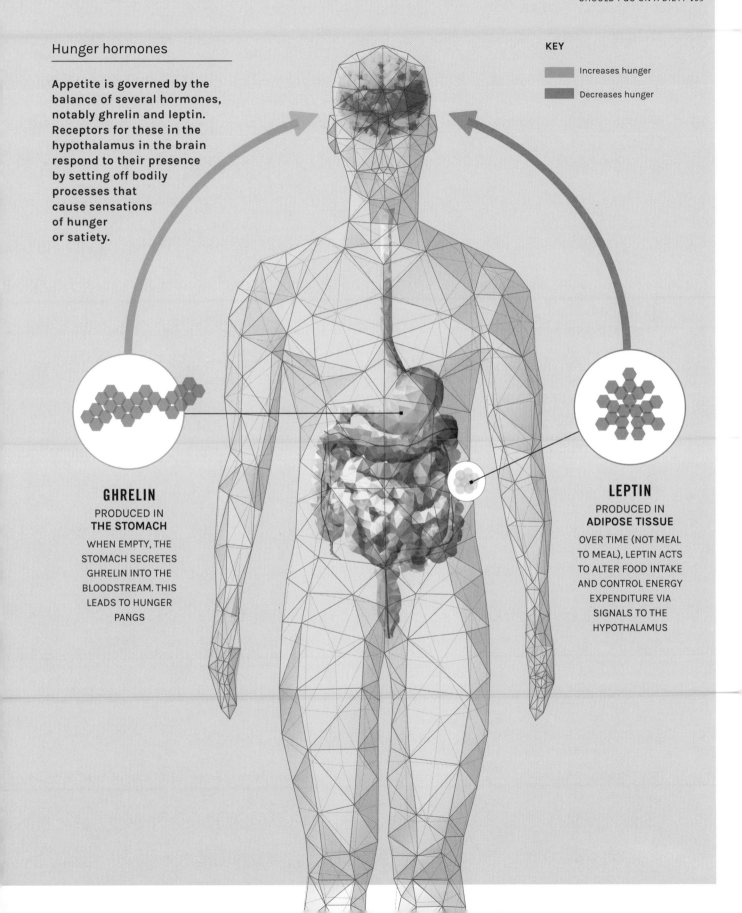

KEY

Increases hunger

Decreases hunger

GHRELIN
PRODUCED IN
THE STOMACH

WHEN EMPTY, THE STOMACH SECRETES GHRELIN INTO THE BLOODSTREAM. THIS LEADS TO HUNGER PANGS

LEPTIN
PRODUCED IN
ADIPOSE TISSUE

OVER TIME (NOT MEAL TO MEAL), LEPTIN ACTS TO ALTER FOOD INTAKE AND CONTROL ENERGY EXPENDITURE VIA SIGNALS TO THE HYPOTHALAMUS

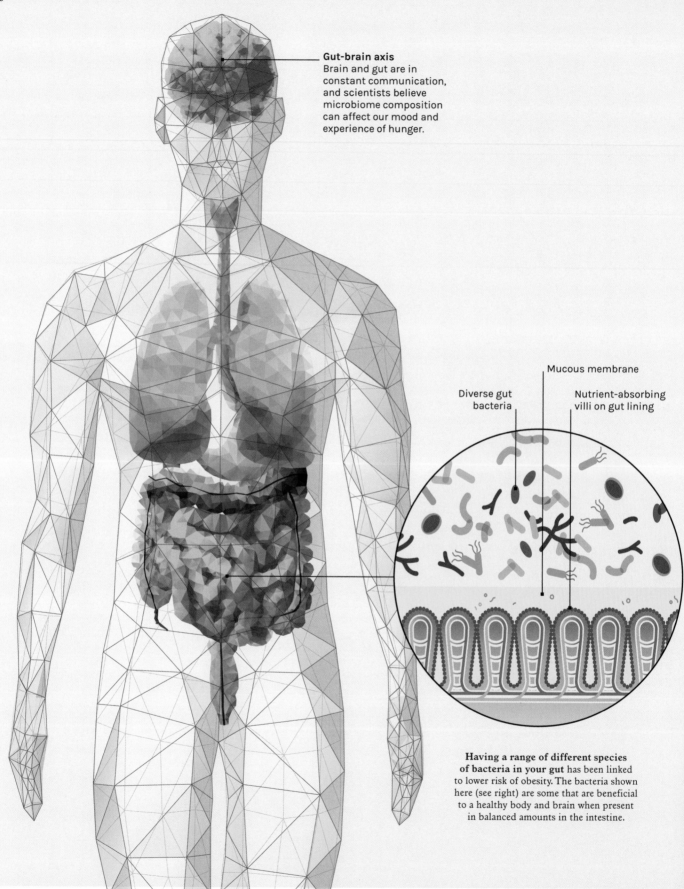

Gut-brain axis
Brain and gut are in constant communication, and scientists believe microbiome composition can affect our mood and experience of hunger.

Mucous membrane

Diverse gut bacteria

Nutrient-absorbing villi on gut lining

Having a range of different species of bacteria in your gut has been linked to lower risk of obesity. The bacteria shown here (see right) are some that are beneficial to a healthy body and brain when present in balanced amounts in the intestine.

CAN MY GUT BACTERIA HELP ME LOSE WEIGHT?

Research suggests that the gut microbiome—the trillions of bacteria that reside in our gut—may be an influential factor in our ability to lose weight.

———————

Fascination with the gut microbiome has grown in recent years, as research has revealed the importance of its diversity on physical and mental health. Gut bacteria are involved in many bodily systems, including immunity, hunger, and digestion (see pages 48–53 and 140–141). Like our genetic makeup, no two people have the same composition of gut bacteria, and studies have uncovered a link between microbiome variation and body composition.

THE IMPACT OF DIVERSITY

One study placed 26 participants on a low-calorie diet rich in fruit and vegetables and found that some people lost more weight than others. Analysis showed this was likely due to a difference in their gut bacteria, which could influence how efficiently food was broken down and thus how much weight was lost. In another study, researchers analyzed the gut bacteria of 169 obese and 123 nonobese adults and found that 23 percent of those who had lower diversity of bacteria were more likely to be obese,

and had increased inflammatory markers, insulin resistance, and lipid levels, all of which increase the risk of diabetes and cardiovascular disease.

Such effects occur because the types and diversity of the bacteria in our microbiome can impact how we process food, as well as other biochemical reactions, thereby influencing weight loss. These differences are likely due to a combination of genetics and environment. For instance, the most heritable bacterial species, *Christensenellaceae*, is found more predominantly in lean people and has been shown to protect against weight gain in rats. We can increase our gut microbiota diversity by consuming a varied, predominantly plant-based diet that is rich in fiber and by trying probiotic fermented foods, as well as limiting our use of unnecessary antibiotics and medications. However, more research is needed to confirm just how much of an impact our gut bacteria can have on weight loss. As yet, there is no definition of what a healthy gut microbiome should look like, beyond diversity.

ENTEROCOCCUS
FAECALIS

AKKERMANSIA
MUCINIPHILA

CHRISTENSENELLA
MINUTA

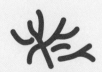

BIFIDO-
BACTERIUM

LACTOBACILLUS

ESCHERICHIA COLI
(HARMLESS
STRAINS)

CAN LIQUID FOODS HELP ME LOSE WEIGHT?

Meal replacement shakes and soups are portion- and calorie-controlled drinks that are consumed in place of meals or snacks in weight-loss programs. These products are often hailed as rapid weight-loss methods, but is there any truth in these claims?

For some, liquid meals help kick-start weight loss, but research suggests they are effective only in the short term. They are not recommended for long-term use. In fact, the potentially tricky return to solid foods increases the chance of weight gain.

THE PROS

Research into liquid meals shows some positive results. Participants who restricted their oral intake to about 800 calories per day on a liquid diet achieved significant weight loss at 12 months. They had foods reintroduced after three to five months and still managed to maintain weight loss. So while liquid diets are unsustainable in the long term, they can help instigate behavior change when people realize that they can lose weight and experience positive benefits to their physical and mental well-being.

Meal-replacement products can be convenient for busy dieters and eliminate decision-making at mealtimes. Additionally, they are often fortified with micronutrients. Some (expensive) brands even claim to be more nutritious than the average meal!

Smoothies can be great on-the-go options. Having the occasional smoothie for breakfast or lunch can be convenient as well as nutritious.

THE CONS

Chewing enhances nutrient absorption. One study found that chewing almonds between 25 and 40 times suppressed hunger and increased the body's ability to absorb nutrients from the almonds. Those who don't chew properly can experience digestive problems and end up snacking more later. The same is true for those relying on liquid meals.

After relying on liquid meals for a period of time and achieving some weight loss, problems can arise when individuals return to eating regular meals. It is very easy to slip into old eating habits and regain the weight. This can be amplified by hormonal changes in the body following dietary restriction and a lowered metabolic rate (see pages 92–93).

Liquid meals can instill a poor relationship with food (see pages 210–211). In addition, following a set diet plan can reduce an individual's ability to respond to internal hunger cues and skew feelings of satiety (see pages 104–105). This can make the transition back to solid food even harder. Lastly, but importantly, liquid meals take the enjoyment and social aspect out of eating. Enjoying meals with family and friends makes a significant contribution to your well-being.

HOMEMADE SOUPS AND SMOOTHIES

There's nothing wrong with liquid foods alongside a balanced diet of solid foods. The odd smoothie isn't such a bad idea. It's an easy way to get a lot of nutrients into your diet, especially if you don't enjoy eating fruits and vegetables (see Nutritious additions, below) or if you've lost your appetite and feel more comfortable drinking than eating.

Make soups with lots of vegetables to add plenty of fiber into your diet.

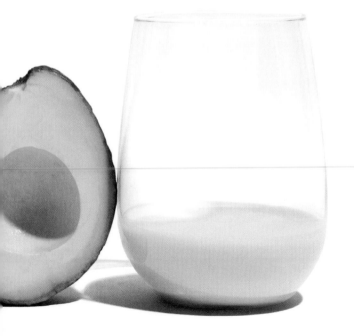

Nutritious additions

WHEN MAKING SMOOTHIES AT HOME, YOU CAN SQUEEZE IN EVEN MORE NUTRITION AND REDUCE YOUR SUGAR INTAKE.

Many smoothies you buy will be fruit heavy. Manufacturers know that the sugars in the fruit make their products more palatable (see page 64). By making your own smoothies, you can increase the vegetable content. Try adding healthy fats, such as flaxseeds and avocado. You could also add some protein powder to help make your nutritious beverage more of a complete meal.

SHOULD I CUT OR REDUCE CARBS?

Low carb diets, like Keto, Atkins, and Paleo, have gained much popularity in recent years, in large part due to the media coverage describing "low-carb" or "no-carb" as the big secret to weight loss. This simply isn't true.

Everyone's carbohydrate needs vary depending on factors like age, sex, build, and activity levels. If you feel you consume more carbs than is right for your body, reducing to bring balance to your diet is sensible. That's not the same as going low-carb.

In the media, and in some scientific literature, carbs are often dismissed as fattening. It's true that society's carbohydrate requirements have reduced due to less active lifestyles, yet carbs remain an important part of a balanced diet. Remember that Japan has one of the lowest obesity rates *and* one of the highest rates of carbohydrate consumption!

FLUID LOSS

Energy from carbs (in the form of glucose) can be converted to glycogen molecules and stored along with the water needed to reconvert it to glucose for future use. On a low-carb diet, the body makes fewer glycogen stores, so the corresponding water is absent. This sudden weight loss is often confused for fat loss.

LOW-CARB DIETS

Low-carb diets advocate the elimination or marked reduction of carbs such as grains (pasta, rice, and breads), starchy fruits and vegetables, and legumes.

The glycogen weight-loss illusion

Each gram of glycogen (stored glucose) is stored with 3g water. The elimination of this water when glycogen stores are depleted on a low-carb diet is often confused for loss of fat.

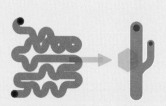

DIGEST CARBS

Carbs are broken down during digestion, releasing glucose into the bloodstream.

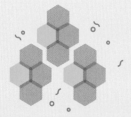

STORE GLYCOGEN

Excess glucose is converted to glycogen and stored in the liver and muscles alongside water, at a ratio of 1 part glycogen to 3 parts water.

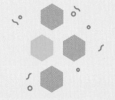

RELEASE GLUCOSE

The water is used to reconvert glycogen to glucose when energy is needed. The glucose is released into the bloodstream along with the water.

Type 2 diabetes

THE ONLY CASE IN WHICH A LOW-CARB DIET HAS PROVEN HEALTH BENEFITS IS THAT OF TYPE 2 DIABETES.
A low-carb diet can be a safe and effective short-term weight-management solution for people with type 2 diabetes who would like to lose weight. It can help improve glycemic control and reduce cardiovascular risk. It's important to have the guidance of a health professional to support any necessary changes to relevant diabetes medications and monitor blood glucose and the risk of hypoglycemia (see pages 170–173).

Studies show there is no significant difference in weight loss between low-carb and low-fat diets. While studies reveal a reduction in weight on the ketogenic diet, it is not sustained long term. These studies have a high dropout rate, showing just how difficult it is to stick to a low-carb diet.

Carbs offer many health benefits (see page 12). If you suddenly restrict them, you may experience headaches and digestive symptoms such as constipation. The fiber in carbs has several benefits, including improving digestion and maintaining blood sugar levels. The keto diet, which excludes many fruits and vegetables, may cause constipation, and keto dieters can miss out on the long-term health benefits of nourishing their gut bacteria (see pages 48–53).

Restricting carbs can cause fatigue, low mood, and cravings. It's not recommended for those recovering from an eating disorder or disordered eating (see pages 210–211), or for children.

MACRONUTRIENT IMBALANCE

Restricting any food group can result in nutritional deficiency. When we remove or restrict carbs, we may turn to other macronutrients to fill the gap. Dietary proteins and fats may increase to unhealthy levels, which may reduce feelings of hunger to help with weight loss but cause other issues such as increased cholesterol. Research found young healthy adults following a low-carb, high-fat diet had a 44 percent increase in LDL ("bad") cholesterol (see page 17). Keto diets encourage foods high in fat, but if you don't differentiate between saturated and unsaturated fats, your LDL cholesterol levels could easily rise, increasing your risk for heart disease and stroke.

CARB REFERENCE INTAKE

225–325g
per day

LOW-CARB DIET

‹130g
per day

KETO DIET

‹50g
per day

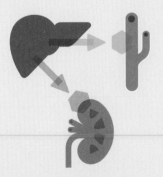

STORES IN LIVER

Glycogen stored in the liver is used first. The water used to convert it to glucose travels via the bloodstream to the kidneys to be expelled as urine.

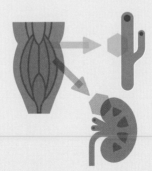

STORES IN MUSCLE

Once the liver's glycogen supply is depleted, the body relies on the glycogen stores in the muscles.

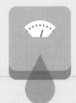

WATER WEIGHT

When you cut carbs, your body depletes glycogen stores, releasing stored water. It's the loss of this, (not fat) that shows on the scales.

WHAT IS A DETOX DIET AND DETOX TEA?

"Detox" is a buzzword in the diet industry. Many products and diet plans promise to rid the body of toxins, help you lose weight, and even reduce cellulite. But detoxes are unnecessary, because your body has a highly effective detoxification system of its own.

The truth is, we don't need to "cleanse" or detox ourselves at all, and following this sort of diet will not have this desired effect.

The idea of feeling clean after a detox diet is what spurs dieters to embark repeatedly on expensive and immensely restrictive detox diets. We come into contact with environmental toxins every single day in the air we breathe and the food we eat, for instance. The body is a wonderful organism, which, through the action of the liver, effectively removes toxins and waste products that make it into the body system.

It is possible that following one of these detox plans may lead to some weight loss, but most of that will be water loss (see pages 110–111) and will be regained when you return to eating normally.

RISKS WITH NO REWARD

Over time, detox diets also give you a greater risk of nutrient deficiencies due to the dietary restrictions they impose. These restrictions may also leave you feeling deprived and probably hungry, which may lead to subsequent overeating.

The bottom line is that detox diets are not good for weight loss and are a serious no-go in terms of nutrition. No health professional would recommend a detox diet because you do not need to detox.

DETOX TEAS

The "teatox" has gained much attention on social media recently, with many people making sensational claims of weight loss. It is entirely possible that you may lose weight in the short term on any new diet regime, but there is no scientific evidence to support the notion that drinking tea will help you lose weight.

Detox teas or "skinny" teas have hit the headlines with claims of being able to help you lose weight fast without dieting by sending your metabolism into overdrive. You can see the allure!

Detoxification by the liver

During digestion, nutrient-laden blood from the small intestine is passed to the liver for processing. Cells in the liver called hepatocytes sift out nutrients and redirect them to wherever they are needed in the body. At the same time, hepatocytes break down toxins and send the waste on to be excreted.

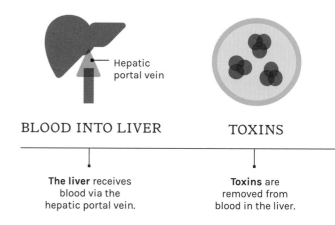

Hepatic portal vein

BLOOD INTO LIVER

TOXINS

The liver receives blood via the hepatic portal vein.

Toxins are removed from blood in the liver.

In reality, teatoxes can be dangerous and are not recommended. Some products are simply laxatives in tea form. The key ingredient is senna, which is used to treat constipation. It irritates the stomach lining to stimulate bowel movements and acts as a diuretic. Using senna can cause dehydration, cramps, and diarrhea and result in inadequate nutrient absorption, causing depletion of key minerals such as calcium, sodium, and potassium.

Regular or prolonged use of senna can damage the gut lining and disrupt electrolyte balance, potentially causing heart damage.

The loss of bulk caused by using a laxative to "clear out" can make you feel and look slimmer in the short term, due to your bowels being abnormally empty. But it has no impact on fat loss, because calories from food are absorbed in your small intestine (see page 28), much further up the digestive tract than the colon, which is where the effect of the laxative is felt. So with skinny teas, you end up spending a fortune on something that, basically, confines you to the toilet!

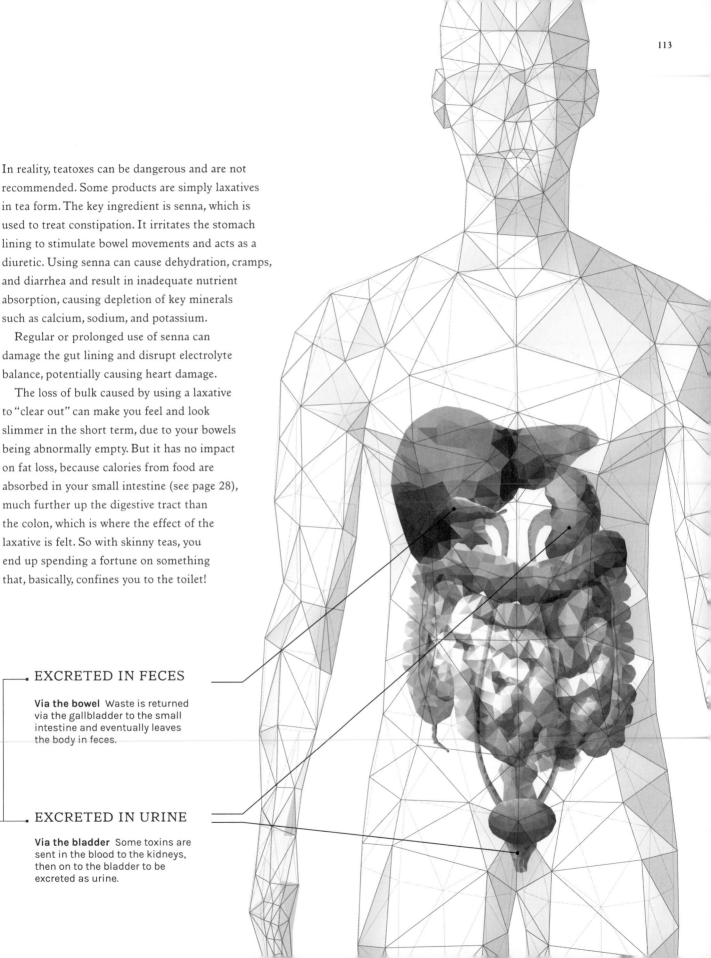

EXCRETED IN FECES

Via the bowel Waste is returned via the gallbladder to the small intestine and eventually leaves the body in feces.

EXCRETED IN URINE

Via the bladder Some toxins are sent in the blood to the kidneys, then on to the bladder to be excreted as urine.

IS IT OK TO SKIP MEALS?

It sounds simple: skip a meal or two here and there, and you will be able to lose weight without having to worry too much about what you're actually eating. But is it that easy—and could it even be potentially harmful?

Intermittent fasting (IF) is a weight-loss method that has grown in popularity in recent years. There are three main types:

● **Whole-day fasting**: this includes the well-known 5:2 diet, with a limited 400–500 calorie intake on two days of the week only.

● **Alternate-day fasting**: on fasted days, it's recommended you eat just one meal.

● **Time-restricted eating**: an example is the 16:8 plan, where you eat the same amount of food as usual, but during an eight-hour window each day. Often, followers opt to skip breakfast.

Most of the research surrounding IF is based on simple calorie restriction. Most likely, these diets are popular because they offer a straightforward way to reduce energy intake that often leads to weight loss. For example, many people following time-restricted eating "fast" while asleep, then eat fewer calories than they normally would because they also have a shorter time period within which to eat. However, IF won't work for everyone, such as those with a tendency to comfort or binge eat, rather than stop when full (see pages 212–213).

Time-restricted eating

This method typically takes advantage of our natural fasting period of sleep by setting an evening cutoff for eating. Here is an example of a daily schedule based on 16 hours of fasting.

GLYCOGEN

DINNER WINDOW

WINDOW CLOSES

EVENING DRINKS

FASTING 0–12 HOURS

6 p.m.:
Window opens
Eat at any time within the two-hour window.

8 p.m.:
Cut-off point
Try not to eat too quickly, even if you are running late.

Any time:
Stay hydrated
Drink water, herbal tea, or tea/coffee without milk; avoid alcohol, fruit juice, or sugar-sweetened drinks.

Energy from glycogen
During this period, the body burns glycogen stored in the liver.

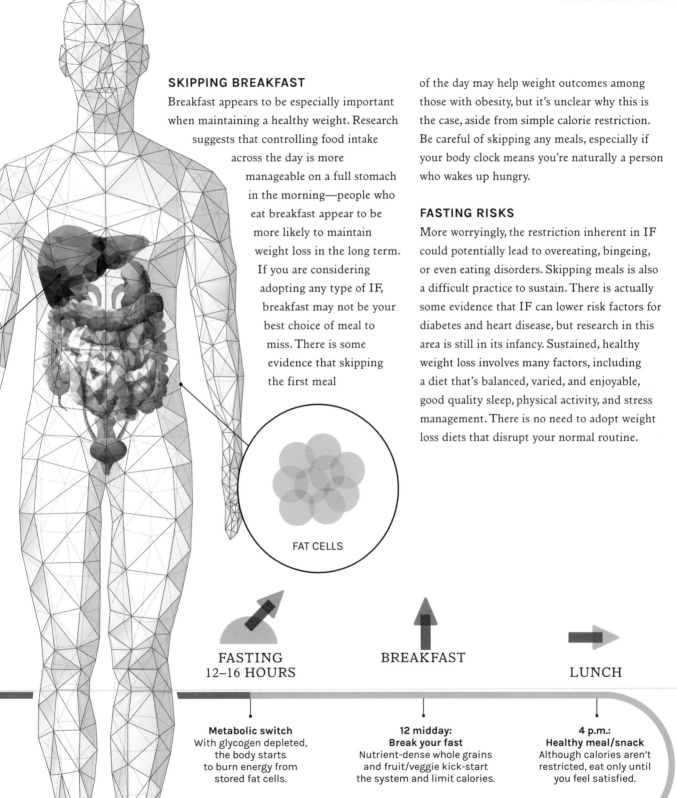

SKIPPING BREAKFAST

Breakfast appears to be especially important when maintaining a healthy weight. Research suggests that controlling food intake across the day is more manageable on a full stomach in the morning—people who eat breakfast appear to be more likely to maintain weight loss in the long term. If you are considering adopting any type of IF, breakfast may not be your best choice of meal to miss. There is some evidence that skipping the first meal of the day may help weight outcomes among those with obesity, but it's unclear why this is the case, aside from simple calorie restriction. Be careful of skipping any meals, especially if your body clock means you're naturally a person who wakes up hungry.

FASTING RISKS

More worryingly, the restriction inherent in IF could potentially lead to overeating, bingeing, or even eating disorders. Skipping meals is also a difficult practice to sustain. There is actually some evidence that IF can lower risk factors for diabetes and heart disease, but research in this area is still in its infancy. Sustained, healthy weight loss involves many factors, including a diet that's balanced, varied, and enjoyable, good quality sleep, physical activity, and stress management. There is no need to adopt weight loss diets that disrupt your normal routine.

FAT CELLS

FASTING
12–16 HOURS

BREAKFAST

LUNCH

Metabolic switch
With glycogen depleted,
the body starts
to burn energy from
stored fat cells.

12 midday:
Break your fast
Nutrient-dense whole grains
and fruit/veggie kick-start
the system and limit calories.

4 p.m.:
Healthy meal/snack
Although calories aren't
restricted, eat only until
you feel satisfied.

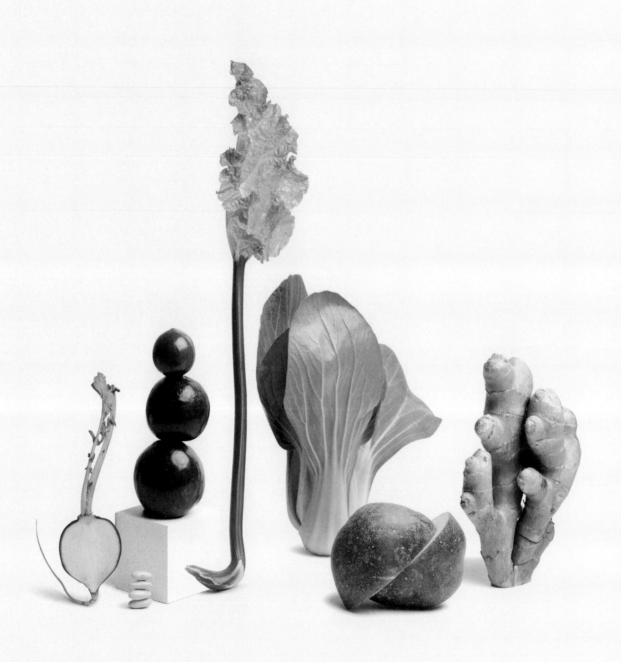

SHOULD I CHOOSE PLANT-BASED NUTRITION?

WHAT DOES PLANT-BASED ACTUALLY MEAN?

"Plant-based" has become a trendy term, but it isn't always clear what exactly people mean by it. Does it mean eating more plants, or just plants? And how does it differ from being vegan or vegetarian?

Plant-based eating is becoming increasingly popular, with a total of 57 percent of US households purchasing plant-based food in 2020, up from 53 percent in 2019. As the trend grows, so do misunderstandings of its original meaning.

As you might expect, a plant-based diet focuses on foods primarily from plants. This includes not only fruits and vegetables but also nuts, seeds, oils, whole grains, and legumes. It doesn't mean that you are vegetarian or vegan and never eat meat or dairy. Instead, you are proportionately choosing more of your foods from plant sources.

A well-planned plant-based diet can support healthy living at every age and life stage. Including a wide variety of healthy whole foods will ensure your diet is balanced and sustainable. However, like all diets, a poorly planned plant-based diet may leave you at risk of certain nutrient deficiencies, which may affect both the mind and body.

VEGANISM

Veganism is more than just a dietary choice; it encompasses a way of life in which the aim is to exclude cruelty to animals in all forms and for sustainability and environmental reasons. This means vegans avoid using animal or animal-derived products in food or clothing or for any other purpose.

It can be very easy to use a product or consume a food that isn't vegan if you don't know what to look for on the label. Animal-derived ingredients crop up in all sorts of places, such as food additives in bread, gelatin products, some fruit juices, and lanolin-derived vitamin D in cereals or supplements (vitamin D2 and lichen-derived vitamin D3 are suitable for vegans).

Veganism is often hailed as a healthy way to live, but it's possible to be an unhealthy vegan. You could keep to a vegan diet yet eat fast foods and processed ready-made meals, use saturated-fat-rich coconut oil in your cooking, and enjoy high-sugar foods such as vegan chocolate brownies. Veganism itself won't necessarily give you the nutrients you need for good health and energy (see pages 130–131).

VEGETARIANISM

Vegetarianism has been around for centuries and is becoming increasingly popular. Vegetarians don't eat fish, meat, or chicken, including stock and fat from animals, insects and gelatin, or animal rennet. A diet can include vegetables and fruits, grains and legumes, nuts and seeds, eggs, dairy products, and honey. There are also a number of different subcategories of vegetarianism:
- **Lacto-ovo vegetarians** eat dairy foods and eggs but not meat, poultry, or seafood.
- **Ovo-vegetarians** include eggs but avoid all other animal foods, including dairy.
- **Lacto-vegetarians** eat dairy foods but exclude eggs, meat, poultry, and seafood.

Ultimately, plant-based eating should be about eating meals with more vegetables and legumes and swapping animal-derived produce for plant protein alternatives such as beans, legumes, and tofu.

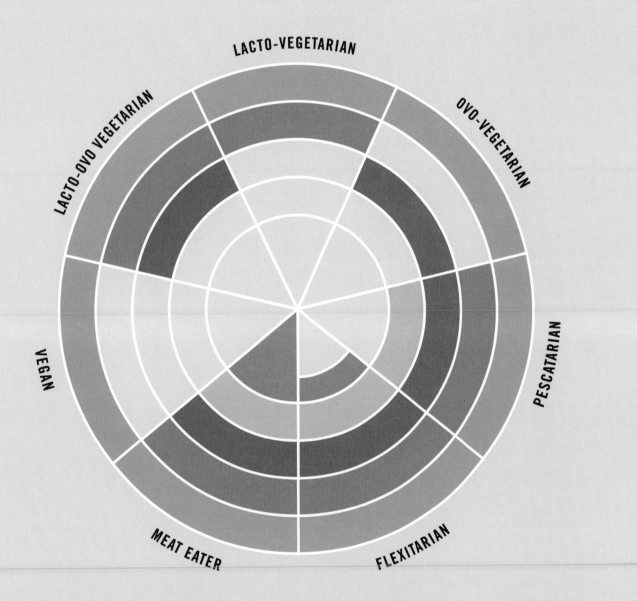

LACTO-VEGETARIAN

OVO-VEGETARIAN

LACTO-OVO VEGETARIAN

PESCATARIAN

VEGAN

MEAT EATER

FLEXITARIAN

Plant-based combinations
Instead of comprising a rigid set of rules, a
plant-based diet can mean a variety of dietary
combinations, including or excluding animal-
derived products as desired but predominantly
featuring foods from plant sources.

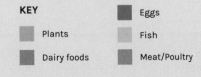

KEY

Plants

Dairy foods

Eggs

Fish

Meat/Poultry

WHAT ARE THE HEALTH BENEFITS OF PLANT-BASED NUTRITION?

The idea that vegetables are good for us is one of the most obvious principles of nutrition. In fact, there are many reasons why increasing the proportion of plants in your diet can improve your health.

There are numerous benefits to following a plant-based diet, including reduced environmental impact and lower costs. There can also be significant health benefits, provided you avoid nutritional deficiencies.

YOUR NUTRITIONAL NEEDS

The dietary guidelines for Americans recommends a diet low in saturated fat and high in whole grains, fresh fruits, and vegetables. If you follow a balanced vegetarian diet based on whole grains, legumes, vegetables, fruits, nuts, and seeds, you should easily exceed the guidelines for eating five portions of fruits or vegetables a day, and your meals will be naturally high in fiber and low in saturated fat.

Things are more complicated when it comes to the essential vitamins and minerals that your body needs on a daily basis, like calcium, iron, omega-3 fatty acids, and iodine, as well as vitamin B12. It is easy to get enough of these when following a omnivorous diet, but some of these nutrients are less "bio-available" in plant-based foods, meaning it is more difficult for the body to use those nutrients

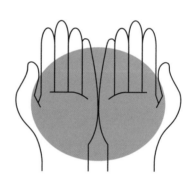

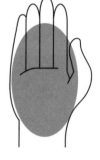

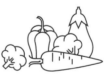

A balanced vegan diet

The key to a healthy vegan diet is making sure all your nutritional needs are met once animal products have been eliminated. This may mean adjusting your intake of certain foods to achieve a varied and balanced mix of protein, fiber, vitamins, minerals, and healthy fats that will leave you feeling energized and strong. Aim to match the daily and weekly amounts recommended here.

2½ CUPS
VEGETABLES

Per day.
Eat as many vegetables as you can, of as many different colors as you can; they are a key source of essential nutrients and fiber.

2 CUPS
FRUIT

Per day.
One portion is about one piece of fruit, such as an apple or banana, or about 3oz (85g). A rich source of dietary fiber, vitamins, minerals, and antioxidants.

when you eat the foods. It is important to make sure you are getting the right amount of protein and micronutrients from your diet (see pages 128–131).

THE POWER OF PLANTS

A lot of research supports the argument that a plant-based diet increases longevity and reduces the risk of certain health conditions. Well-balanced plant-based diets that are low in saturated fats can contribute toward managing a healthy weight, reducing your risk of type 2 diabetes, cardiovascular disease, and even some cancers. There is also a lot of evidence that points toward reduced blood pressure when omitting animal products from our diets.

Fiber is an important factor in why plant-based eating is beneficial to health. Eating a variety of plant-based foods may help you get the recommended 28g of fiber each day, which supports the gut microbiome. Prebiotic foods (see pages 52–53), including garlic, leeks, bananas, and oats, are particularly effective in this regard. Studies show that eating a high-fiber diet can lead to better control of blood-sugar levels and cholesterol levels, too. And fiber from whole grains has also been linked to a reduced risk of developing several diseases, including type 2 diabetes.

There are healthy and happy people who eat animal products and healthy and happy people who eat only plants. By reducing meat, fish, and dairy to minimal amounts and increasing plant-based alternatives, you can get the best of both worlds and lessen your environmental impact. While this approach does not address the ethical concerns associated with animal products, it may be a huge step for someone who consumes meat, fish, and dairy daily in their diet.

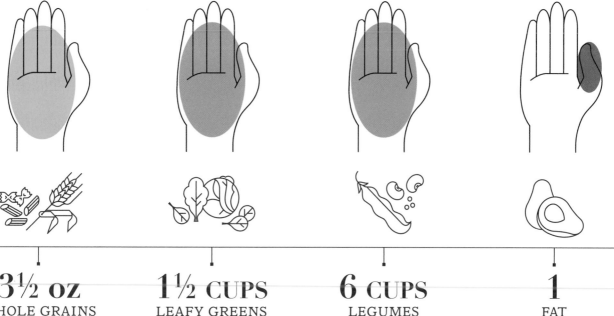

3½ OZ
WHOLE GRAINS

Per day.
One portion is about 1oz (30g) of grain or a slice of whole wheat bread. Choose brown rice, whole wheat pasta, quinoa, buckwheat, barley, farro, and sprouted grains for protein and fiber.

1½ CUPS
LEAFY GREENS

Per week.
One portion is about 3oz (85g) of leafy green vegetables such as broccoli, cabbage, kale, and spinach, which are packed with vitamins, minerals, and antioxidants.

6 CUPS
LEGUMES

Per week.
One portion is about 125g of beans, peas, or lentils, which are high in protein and low in fat, and contain no cholesterol.

1
FAT

Per day.
About 1oz (27g) of oil or nuts, or half an avocado. High-fat whole foods, as well as dairy substitutes like soy and almond, are a healthy source of fat but should be kept to a single portion.

IS PLANT-BASED ALWAYS HEALTHIER?

The benefits of a primarily plant-based diet, while good, are dependent on whether it is followed for optimal health. Without careful choices, plant-based has the potential to be full of unhealthy items and there is a risk of nutritional deficiencies.

Debates over our diets are often highly emotive. The conversation around plant-based eating often focuses on personal preference and environmental and ethical concerns, while nutritional science gets left behind.

FIND THE RIGHT BALANCE

The nutritional benefits of eating more plants are grounded in solid evidence. A diverse range of plant foods providing 28g of fiber each day supports gut health, while fruits and vegetables are great sources for a range of vitamins and minerals.

However, some plant-based diets risk not getting the right nutrition through protein, vitamin, and mineral intake. These risks can be overcome by choosing the right vegetarian foods and, when necessary, supplements (see pages 128–131).

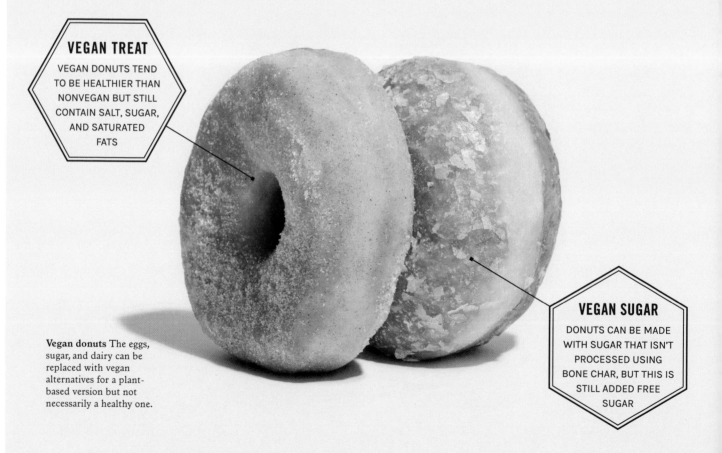

VEGAN TREAT
VEGAN DONUTS TEND TO BE HEALTHIER THAN NONVEGAN BUT STILL CONTAIN SALT, SUGAR, AND SATURATED FATS

VEGAN SUGAR
DONUTS CAN BE MADE WITH SUGAR THAT ISN'T PROCESSED USING BONE CHAR, BUT THIS IS STILL ADDED FREE SUGAR

Vegan donuts The eggs, sugar, and dairy can be replaced with vegan alternatives for a plant-based version but not necessarily a healthy one.

For example, soy, quinoa, and nuts are good sources of protein, and tofu, lentils, and spinach are good sources of iron. But some nutrients are trickier to get. Iodine, for instance, is mostly found in dairy products and fish. The iodine content of plant foods depends on the iodine content of the soil, which is variable. Foods grown closer to the ocean tend to be higher in iodine. Where soils are iodine deficient, iodized salt and seaweed can provide iodine.

The way vegetables are cooked is also relevant: steamed vegetables are far more nutritious than deep-fried, for instance. And a lot of plant-based alternatives to animal products are not nutritionally balanced. For example, pulled pork is often replaced by jackfruit, but the latter contains no protein. There are also many vegan processed foods available that are unhealthy—vegetarian sausage rolls, for instance, can be high in salt and saturated fat.

QUESTIONS TO BE ANSWERED

Contrary to what most research suggests, there is some research indicating that plant-based diets may contribute to cardiovascular disease. A two-decade UK-based study of 50,000 people analyzed the risk of stroke and other health problems based on diet. The researchers found that, compared with meat eaters, rates of heart disease (such as angina or heart attack) were 13 percent lower in pescatarians and 22 percent lower in vegetarians. But the results also showed that rates of stroke were 20 percent higher among vegetarians. This was mostly due to

hemorrhagic stroke (bleeding into the brain), and was not observed among pescatarians.

Studies like this may sound groundbreaking, but it's important to check their limitations. The overall risk of stroke in vegetarians was small, equal to 3 extra cases per 1,000 people over 10 years. What's more, this particular study was observational, meaning the researchers did not account for other relevant variables besides diet.

There are many other factors to consider, but the more robust research suggests that plant-based diets, if conducted well, can be a healthy way of eating and that meat eaters don't have to give up meat to be healthier—they can simply reduce it.

The "Anti-nutrient"

PHYTIC ACID IS PRESENT IN PLANT SEEDS SUCH AS NUTS, WHOLE GRAINS, AND BEANS.
In the body, the acid binds to minerals to form phytate, which is known as an "anti-nutrient" since it impairs the absorption of zinc, iron, and calcium and can cause deficiencies in those on a plant-based diet. As an antioxidant that can help prevent cardiovascular disease and kidney stones, however, it also has health benefits, so avoiding these foods is not advised. Soaking, cooking, fermenting, and sprouting beans and grains will reduce their phytate content, while the minerals affected can also be sourced elsewhere: zinc in tofu; iron in dates and strawberries; calcium in leafy greens.

HOW CAN I EAT IN A SUSTAINABLE WAY?

Many people have this question on their minds at the moment, but it can be difficult to understand the issues involved. Be reassured that there are practical steps you can take with your diet to minimize your environmental impact.

It is more important than ever before that we take care of planet Earth. How we use natural resources for food production must become more sustainable for the sake of future generations and for overall harmony of life on the planet.

The agriculture industry is the biggest driver of biodiversity vons (GHGe). Fossil fuels are used all along supply chains and beyond, from farming and production to distribution and delivery to waste disposal. We all have the power to make dietary changes, large or small, to contribute to solutions.

EAT LESS MEAT AND DAIRY

If you eat meat, you don't need to give it up completely. Consider reducing your consumption of red meat to one portion per week. This change alone could make a difference.

Half of the habitable land on the planet is used for agriculture, with 77 percent of it dedicated to rearing livestock. Yet meat and dairy produce provide only 17 percent of global energy intake, and only 33 percent of global protein intake. This resource-intensive approach to food production isn't paying off, either in terms of nutrition or sustainability.

Meat and dairy production are responsible for two-thirds of the GHGe of the US's food industry. Globally, countless ecosystems are destroyed to make space for grazing livestock or for raising feed crops for them. At this point, even the most dedicated meat eaters are choosing to lean more on plant-based sources of protein as a lifeline for the planet. Going plant-based doesn't mean eating no meat whatsoever. Try following the planetary diet (see page 127) as closely as possible. There are many

Producing protein sources This chart compares the use of resources and the GHGe involved in the production of a 3.5oz (100g) portion of protein from various food sources. It shows that producing plant sources such as peas and tofu has considerably less impact than sheep meat or cheese.

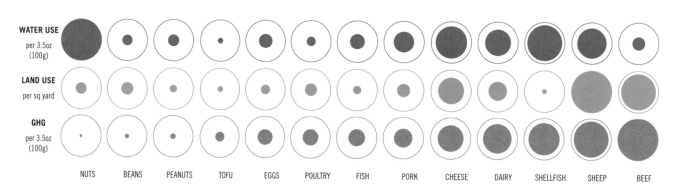

	NUTS	BEANS	PEANUTS	TOFU	EGGS	POULTRY	FISH	PORK	CHEESE	DAIRY	SHELLFISH	SHEEP	BEEF
WATER USE per 3.5oz (100g)													
LAND USE per sq yard													
GHG per 3.5oz (100g)													

ways of using plant-based proteins (see pages 128–129). Educate yourself on the key nutrients you need to include on a plant-based diet (see pages 130–131).

THINK LOGISTICS

Shopping locally and seasonally where possible will reduce the length of the supply chains involved in the food you eat, thereby reducing emissions. Do what you can to reduce food waste. Plan meals and snacks for the week ahead and shop accordingly to help you avoid buying excess perishable produce.

If you have produce that's about to spoil, think about freezing it. Blanch vegetables and fruit before freezing them. Or cook up meals to freeze in portions for your later convenience.

Try growing your own, then pick just what you need. Herbs on a windowsill, a sack of potatoes on the back doorstep, or a patch of garden dedicated to vegetables is good for body, mind, soul, and planet.

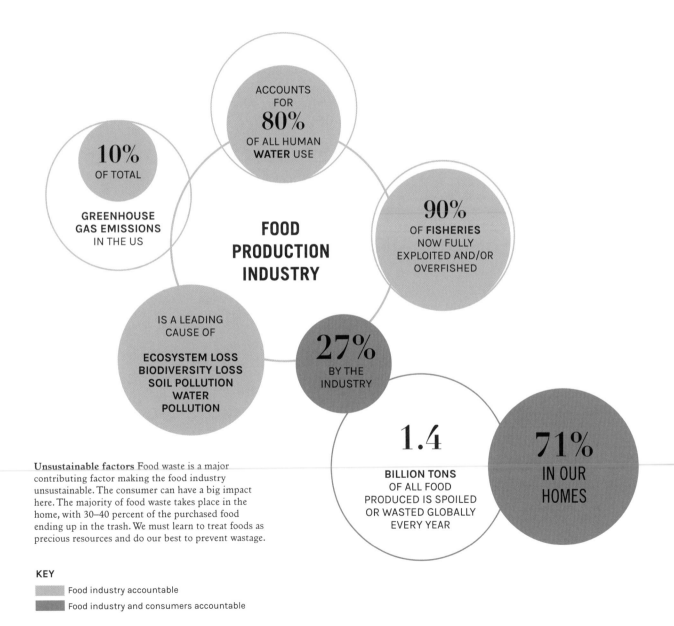

10%
OF TOTAL

**GREENHOUSE
GAS EMISSIONS**
IN THE US

ACCOUNTS
FOR
80%
OF ALL HUMAN
WATER USE

**FOOD
PRODUCTION
INDUSTRY**

90%
OF **FISHERIES**
NOW FULLY
EXPLOITED AND/OR
OVERFISHED

IS A LEADING
CAUSE OF

**ECOSYSTEM LOSS
BIODIVERSITY LOSS
SOIL POLLUTION
WATER
POLLUTION**

27%
BY THE
INDUSTRY

1.4

BILLION TONS
OF ALL FOOD
PRODUCED IS SPOILED
OR WASTED GLOBALLY
EVERY YEAR

71%
IN OUR
HOMES

Unsustainable factors Food waste is a major contributing factor making the food industry unsustainable. The consumer can have a big impact here. The majority of food waste takes place in the home, with 30–40 percent of the purchased food ending up in the trash. We must learn to treat foods as precious resources and do our best to prevent wastage.

KEY

Food industry accountable

Food industry and consumers accountable

IS PLANT-BASED BETTER FOR THE ENVIRONMENT?

Yes, definitely—although not all plant proteins are equal. To make the greatest impact with your plant-based dietary choices, it's important to know which products have the smallest carbon footprint.

When you factor in the impact of the meat and dairy industry (see page 124), a plant-based diet is inarguably the way forward. But most plant products have the edge over others. For instance, soy, a legume, fixes nitrogen into the soil as it grows, reducing the need for nitrogen fertilizers. These produce nitrous oxide, a potent greenhouse gas that leaks into waterways, causing damage to marine life and ecosystems. Soy also has a good nutritional profile, so leaning toward soy products alongside beans and lentils (for balance) is a sound environmental and nutritional choice.

Mycoprotein, an excellent protein source, is often mistakenly considered an unhealthy processed food.

It is a plant-based food made from fungus and produced through fermentation. (You might recognize it by the brand name Quorn.) It has a significantly smaller carbon footprint than animal proteins and uses 90 per ent less land, making it a highly sustainable protein source.

FACTORING WATER USAGE

Water is becoming more scarce, especially in countries that produce most of our foods. The food industry accounts for 70 percent of water use.

This is an important point to consider when using nuts as a protein source. The country of origin and

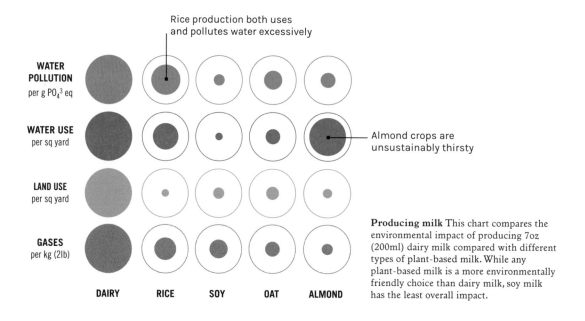

Rice production both uses and pollutes water excessively

WATER POLLUTION
per g PO_4^3 eq

WATER USE
per sq yard

Almond crops are unsustainably thirsty

LAND USE
per sq yard

GASES
per kg (2lb)

DAIRY   RICE   SOY   OAT   ALMOND

Producing milk This chart compares the environmental impact of producing 7oz (200ml) dairy milk compared with different types of plant-based milk. While any plant-based milk is a more environmentally friendly choice than dairy milk, soy milk has the least overall impact.

Planetary diet proportions

Deprivation is not part of the planetary diet. Proportions of food groups are designed with the health of the planet and human nutrition in mind. No food groups are excluded, but the emphasis is on plant-based eating and moderation.

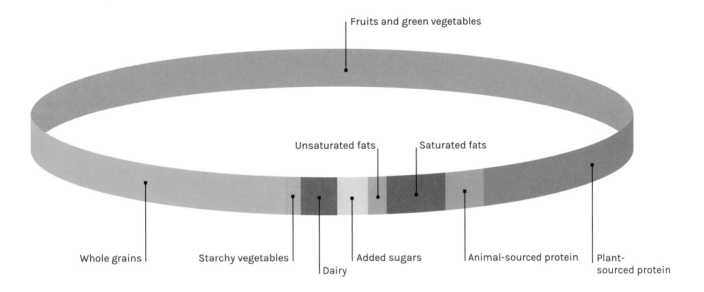

Fruits and green vegetables

Unsaturated fats

Saturated fats

Whole grains

Starchy vegetables

Dairy

Added sugars

Animal-sourced protein

Plant-sourced protein

level of water stress caused by production are relevant. For instance, the production of Californian almonds is exceptionally water inefficient, using around 1.3 gallons of water per almond (Californian farmers have committed to reduce water usage).

THE PLANETARY DIET

The planetary diet is a useful practical guideline for helping you eat sustainably and can be adapted to meet a broad range of dietary needs and cultural preferences. This approach to balancing the diet takes into account both the environmental impact of food production and the nutritional requirements of the human body. The focus is on whole produce, with half of the diet coming from vegetables and fruits. The other half consists primarily of whole grains and plant proteins (beans and lentils) but also includes fats, modest amounts of meat and dairy, and some added sugars and starchy vegetables.

Different from a vegan or vegetarian diet, the planetary diet simply requires you to reduce the number of portions of meat you consume and get the bulk of your protein from plant sources. For red meat fans, you're looking at a burger a week or a large steak a month. Or you could have a couple of portions of chicken and the same of fish per week.

WILL I STRUGGLE TO EAT ENOUGH PROTEIN ON A VEGAN DIET?

It's a misconception that anyone adopting a vegan lifestyle will struggle to get enough protein. Plant proteins may be arranged differently from those in meat and fish, but a sufficiently varied vegan diet will supply more than enough to meet daily needs.

Protein is present in every cell and is fundamental for tissue repair, muscle growth, and more. The idea that a vegan diet is protein deficient derives from the fact that not all protein is "complete." Protein's building blocks are 20 amino acids, and the body has to obtain nine of these from diet; complete protein contains similar amounts of all nine. While meat, eggs, fish, and dairy provide complete protein, most plant-based foods are incomplete. For example, white and brown rice are high in methionine and low in lysine, which is found in many pulses. So vegans should consume as many foods as possible.

Previous research suggested it is necessary to combine incomplete proteins at each meal; now we know eating a mixture over the day is effective, because of how the liver stores amino acids. Also, the body can efficiently use up to only 20g–40g of protein at a time. Healthy adults should eat at least 0.8g per 2lb (1kg) of body weight daily—more, depending on activity levels (see pages 80–81).

PROTEIN SOURCES

Soy-based foods provide complete protein. **Tofu** (8g per 3.5oz) is the best known, while **tempeh** (18g) is a fermented meat substitute with a stronger flavor; soy-based milk and yogurt alternatives are also fermented. Other meat substitutes are **mycoprotein** (see opposite) and high-protein **seitan** (75g), which is made from wheat gluten so may not suit those with an intolerance.

Quinoa (4.4g per 3.5oz) is another complete protein source. It is actually a seed from the

DAILY AVERAGE PROTEIN CONSUMPTION BY REGION

Bar chart showing regions: INDIA, ASIA, AFRICA, S. AMERICA, CHINA, EUROPE, N. AMERICA. Vertical axis from 60g (top) to 0 to 60g (bottom), marked at 10-unit intervals.

KEY

Plant-based protein

Animal-based protein

 Recommended intake

Protein intake: Outside of Europe and North America, it is normal for plants to provide the major source of protein.

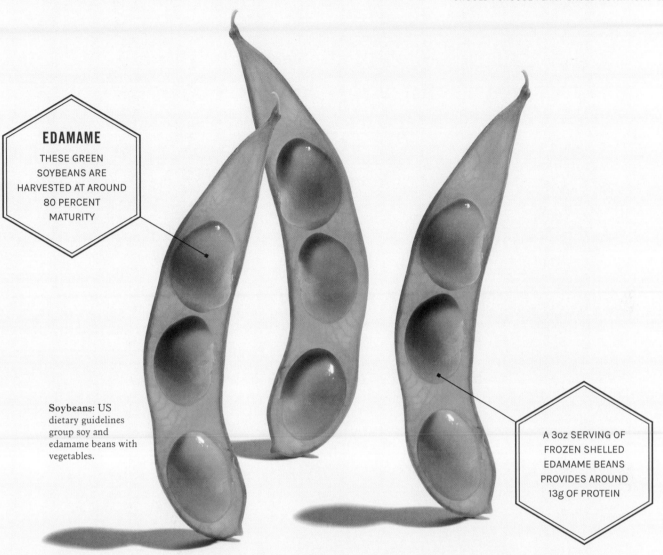

EDAMAME
THESE GREEN
SOYBEANS ARE
HARVESTED AT AROUND
80 PERCENT
MATURITY

Soybeans: US
dietary guidelines
group soy and
edamame beans with
vegetables.

A 3oz SERVING OF
FROZEN SHELLED
EDAMAME BEANS
PROVIDES AROUND
13g OF PROTEIN

Chenopodium quinoa plant, although it's usually grouped with whole grains.

Otherwise, **nuts** and **seeds** are ideal for snacking, in salad or cereal, or in nut butters. They can contain up to 20g of protein per 3.5oz; a portion is around 1oz. **Beans** and **lentils** typically contain about 20g of protein per 3.5oz; one portion is around 4oz cooked. **Fortified foods** like vegan energy balls, breakfast cereals, and protein bars often have soy added. Check labels—"vegan" doesn't mean a food is low in salt, sugar, and fat. Some **vegetables** also provide protein, for example, 2.8g per 3.5oz of broccoli.

What is mycoprotein?

**MYCOPROTEIN IS A MEAT SUBSTITUTE
BETTER KNOWN AS QUORN.**

Its main ingredient, *Fusarium venenatum*, is a microfungus that occurs naturally in soil—fungi aren't classified as plants because they lack chlorophyll and have a different cellular structure. It is fed with carbohydrate in large fermenters and the liquid is separated by centrifugal force to create mycoprotein dough. A complete protein source (11g per 3.5oz), it also contains various micronutrients.

WHAT OTHER NUTRIENTS SHOULD PLANT-BASED EATERS CONSIDER?

Anyone who eats only certain animal-derived foods, or excludes them completely, should still be able to get most of the nutrients they need from a plant-based diet. In some cases, though, it may be necessary to supplement.

Most nutrients are abundant in a plant-based diet. Protein is often a concern but shouldn't be a problem, whereas a vitamin D supplement is necessary for everyone in winter (see pages 138–139). These are some key micronutrients to consider.

As well as ensuring strong bones and teeth, **calcium** regulates muscle contractions and helps blood clot normally. Dairy is a key source; only some plants contain calcium, at fairly low levels.

Even mild **iodine** deficiency can harm a baby's developing brain. It also affects levels of thyroid hormones, which support metabolic function. Plant sources are scarce, so those at higher risk, in particular pregnant or breastfeeding women, should consider supplementing. Talk to your doctor first.

Heart and brain-friendly **omega-3 fatty acids** can be obtained only from diet (see pages 16–17). ALA (alpha-linolenic-acid) is available in various plant sources, but research indicates plants are less effective sources of eicosapentaenoic (EPA) and docosahexaenoic (DHA) acids. EPA and DHA can be taken as microalgae-based supplements.

Vitamin B12 keeps nerve and blood cells healthy. Most plant-based sources can't be processed by the body, although you can sprinkle nutritional yeast on meals or take a daily supplement. Ask your primary care physician to periodically check your B12 levels.

Iron helps maintain the immune system and form hemoglobin, which transports oxygen around the body. Deficiency can lead to anemia (below-average intake is prevalent among young children and women of reproductive age). Vitamin C aids iron absorption.

The body doesn't make **zinc**, which helps make cells and enzymes and processes fat, protein, and carbohydrates; 30g of hemp or pumpkin seeds provides a third of daily adult needs.

CALCIUM	VITAMIN D	IODINE	OMEGA-3
RDA (AGE 19–64): 700mg	**RDA** (VARIES): 8.5mcg–10mcg	**RDA** (ADULTS): 140mcg	**RDA** N/A
PLANT SOURCES DRIED FRUIT | NUTS | TOFU LEAFY GREENS | KIDNEY BEANS | TAHINI	**PLANT SOURCES** OILY FISH | FORTIFIED FOODS UV-EXPOSED MUSHROOOMS	**PLANT SOURCES** FORTIFIED PLANT MILK	**PLANT SOURCES** WALNUTS | HEMP/CHIA SEEDS | FLAXSEED SOY | CANOLA OIL

A SINGLE
BELL PEPPER CAN
PROVIDE MORE THAN
THREE TIMES YOUR
DAILY VITAMIN C
REQUIREMENT

Eat a rainbow: Vitamin C in orange, red, and yellow peppers, and leafy green vegetables and tomatoes, helps absorb more iron within a vegan diet.

Most adults don't consume enough **selenium** (see below). It helps with reproductive health, immune system maintenance, and tissue repair; 2–3 Brazil nuts supply the complete daily requirement.

OXALATES AND PHYTATES

While plant foods are healthy, some can have less beneficial elements—another reason to eat a wide variety. For example, spinach and Swiss chard contain oxalates, an acid that reduces calcium absorption. Various beans, whole grain cereals, nuts, and seeds (including almonds, sesame seeds, and lentils) contain compounds called phytates, which inhibit zinc and iron absorption. Soaking before eating, or adding berries to your cereal, can help.

ORANGE, RED,
AND YELLOW PEPPERS
ARE RIPENED VERSIONS
OF GREEN AND ALL HAVE
VARYING LEVELS OF
MICRONUTRIENTS

VITAMIN B12

RDA
(AGE 19-64): 1.5mcg

PLANT SOURCES
NUTRITIONAL YEAST |
FORTIFIED CEREALS | YEAST
SPREAD

IRON

RDA: MEN 18+ 8.7mg
WOMEN 18+ 14.8mg/50+ 8.7mg

PLANT SOURCES
WHOLE WHEAT | BEANS
LENTILS | PRUNES | DATES
STRAWBERRIES

ZINC

RDA (19-64):
MEN 9.5g
WOMEN 7mg

PLANT SOURCES
NUTS | LENTILS
TOFU | QUINOA

SELENIUM

RDA (19-64):
MEN 75mcg
WOMEN 60mcg

PLANT SOURCES
BRAZIL NUTS | WHOLE WHEAT
BREAD | BROWN RICE | LENTILS

WHY IS IT IMPORTANT TO INCREASE PLANT-BASED DIVERSITY?

There is a lot of buzz around the subject of gut health these days, in particular the positive impact a diverse plant-based diet can have on the gut. This isn't just a health fad—there's good research to support it.

It is widely accepted that we have a healthier gut if we have a diverse range of different gut bacteria, which carry out many important functions that benefit our health. In the gut, we have trillions of microorganisms that are collectively referred to as the gut microbiota (see pages 48–49). What we eat affects the composition of these bacteria.

Research shows that greater gut microbe diversity is associated with better health. One study of over 10,000 stool samples found that those who eat more than 30 types of plant-based foods per week had more diverse gut microbes than those eating less than 10.

A large study of more than 20,000 people found a strong association between a diet high in plant foods and bowel movement frequency. Chronic constipation can have a serious negative effect on your health, so staying "regular" is another benefit of being on a largely plant-based diet.

EXPERIMENTATION AND FAMILIARITY

Consuming a diverse plant-based diet helps you increase your microbiota diversity. Aim to eat more fruits and vegetables than you normally do—most people don't get enough. Experiment with beans and legumes you don't usually use. Remember that plant-based includes whole grains, nuts, and seeds.

When it comes to your macronutrient requirements (see page 10), become familiar with the types of plant-based protein, fat, and carbohydrate sources available. Plant-based carbs can be an excellent source of fiber (see pages 18 and 44), which is important for feeding and maintaining your microbiota.

Plant-based proteins can be combined to provide your full protein requirements (see pages 14–15). Aim to include a variety of fruits and vegetables in your diet. Don't opt for the same things every day.

EAT SEASONALLY

SEASONAL PRODUCE CAN PROVIDE A HIGHER YIELD OF NUTRIENTS. TRY BOOKING A REGULAR DELIVERY WITH A LOCAL FARM TO HELP YOU TRY OUT NEW VEGETABLES

SPREADS AND DIPS

USE THESE REGULARLY AS ADDITIONAL SOURCES OF FIBER, PROTEIN, AND NUTRIENTS. TRY NUT BUTTERS, HUMMUS, SALSAS, AVOCADO DIP, AND BABA GANOUSH

FERMENTED FOODS

FERMENTED FOODS CONTAINING LIVE MICROBES CONTRIBUTE TO THE GUT MICROBIOTA AND CONTAIN PLENTY OF USEFUL NUTRIENTS

Think switch

The only way to increase your plant-based repertoire is to explore alternatives. This doesn't have to be an onerous task. Simply choose one new alternative to try, then incorporate that regularly into your diet before trying another switch.

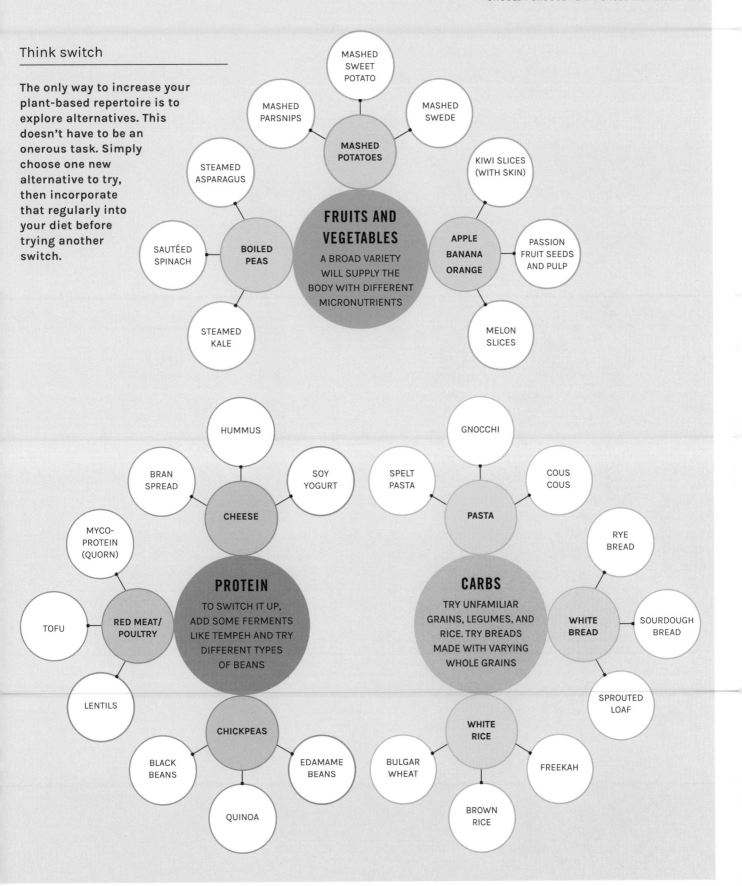

FRUITS AND VEGETABLES
A BROAD VARIETY WILL SUPPLY THE BODY WITH DIFFERENT MICRONUTRIENTS

MASHED SWEET POTATO
MASHED PARSNIPS
MASHED SWEDE
MASHED POTATOES
STEAMED ASPARAGUS
KIWI SLICES (WITH SKIN)
APPLE BANANA ORANGE
PASSION FRUIT SEEDS AND PULP
BOILED PEAS
SAUTÉED SPINACH
STEAMED KALE
MELON SLICES

PROTEIN
TO SWITCH IT UP, ADD SOME FERMENTS LIKE TEMPEH AND TRY DIFFERENT TYPES OF BEANS

HUMMUS
BRAN SPREAD
SOY YOGURT
CHEESE
MYCO-PROTEIN (QUORN)
TOFU
RED MEAT/ POULTRY
LENTILS
CHICKPEAS
BLACK BEANS
EDAMAME BEANS
QUINOA

CARBS
TRY UNFAMILIAR GRAINS, LEGUMES, AND RICE. TRY BREADS MADE WITH VARYING WHOLE GRAINS

GNOCCHI
SPELT PASTA
COUS COUS
PASTA
RYE BREAD
WHITE BREAD
SOURDOUGH BREAD
SPROUTED LOAF
WHITE RICE
BULGAR WHEAT
FREEKAH
BROWN RICE

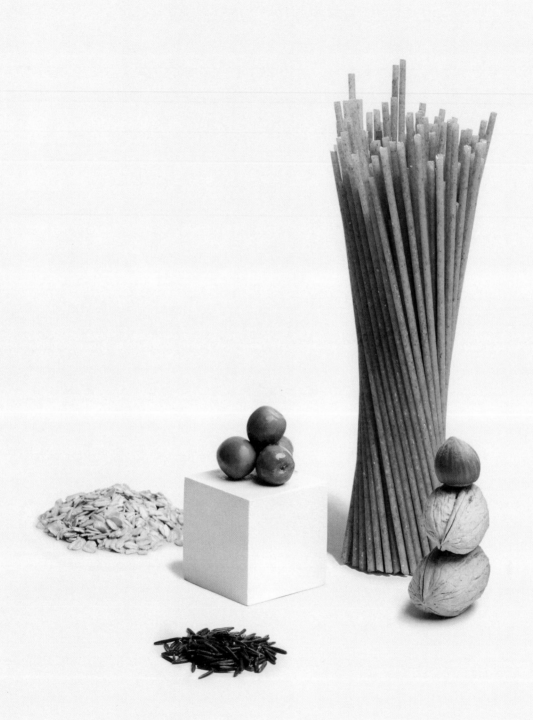

CAN WE EAT FOR BETTER HEALTH OUTCOMES?

CAN I EAT TO BOOST IMMUNITY?

The immune system is incredibly complex and acts like a surveillance system to recognize and respond to pathogens such as bacteria, viruses, and toxins. Our food choices could help, or hinder, its ability to defend the body.

———

"Boosting" immunity is a marketing concept to promote supplements; in fact, our immune system is programmed to work in a highly specific way. Diet can support it to function at its best when under attack and to maintain a protective barrier.

Our immune system is always "on," but when activated, it needs additional energy to fuel the creation of millions of new immune cells to fight the threat. Poor diet can contribute to weakened immune response, as can gut health and antibiotic use (see pages 140–141). Healthy adults should be able to obtain enough of the micronutrients that support immune function from a balanced and varied diet. Plant-based eaters may need to supplement certain nutrients (see pages 130–131); otherwise, it shouldn't be necessary unless medically advised and could even cause health problems. If you feel your immune system isn't working well, or you eat a restricted diet, talk to your primary care physician (PCP).

KEY MICRONUTRIENTS

Aim to regularly eat foods containing these vitamins and minerals. (RDAs are based on US guidelines.)
● Vitamin A supports production of immune cells; a deficiency can increase susceptibility to infections. (RDA age 14–51+: men 900mcg RAE, women 700mcg RAE)
● Vitamin B6 is involved in producing immune cells and processing of antibodies. B9 (folate) and B12 are important for red blood cell function; B12 is also involved in immune cell synthesis. Vegans may need to supplement B12. (RDA: B6, men age 14–50: 1.3mg, age 51+: 1.7mg; women age 14–18: 1.2mg, age 19–50: 1.3mg, age 51+: 1.5mg; Folate,

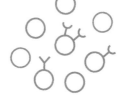

The immune response

———

Two key immune responses work together. The natural response quickly tries to stop the pathogen from spreading, while the slower adaptive response requires exposure to the pathogen first then learns to identify it rapidly.

WHITE BLOOD CELLS

Different types of white blood cells patrol or wait to be alerted. Many types play a role in both stages of the immune response.

PATHOGEN DETECTED

One/more of these cell types detect a pathogen via its antigen (surface protein). They multiply and signal other immune cells.

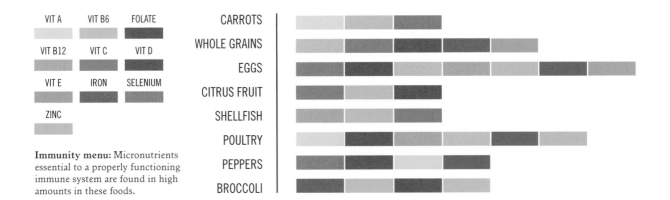

VIT A   VIT B6   FOLATE

VIT B12   VIT C   VIT D

VIT E   IRON   SELENIUM

ZINC

Immunity menu: Micronutrients essential to a properly functioning immune system are found in high amounts in these foods.

CARROTS
WHOLE GRAINS
EGGS
CITRUS FRUIT
SHELLFISH
POULTRY
PEPPERS
BROCCOLI

age 14–19+: 400mcg DFE; B12, age 14–19+: 2.4mcg)

• Vitamin C protects cells and maintains skin, bones, and blood vessels. There's conflicting evidence on whether it reduces the risk of catching viruses. (RDA age 19+: men 40mg, women 75mg)

• Vitamin D deficiency has been linked with a reduced immune response (see pages 138–139).

• Vitamin E deficiency is linked to an increased susceptibility to infection. (RDA age14+: 15mg)

• Iron is important for immune cells; a low level also increases the risk of anemia. Meat-derived iron is easier to absorb than plant-based iron from tofu, beans, and nuts. Vegans and women who lose iron during periods may need to supplement and should consult their PCP. (RDA: men age 19–51+: 8mg; women age 19–50: 18mg, age 51+: 8mg)

• Selenium supports the production of immune cells; within a plant-based diet, 2–3 Brazil nuts daily can provide a sufficient amount. (RDA age 19–64: men 75mcg, women 60mcg)

• Zinc helps produce new immune cells. Deficiency increases susceptibility to respiratory infection. (RDA men age 14+: 11mg; women age 14–18 9mg, age 19+ 8mg)

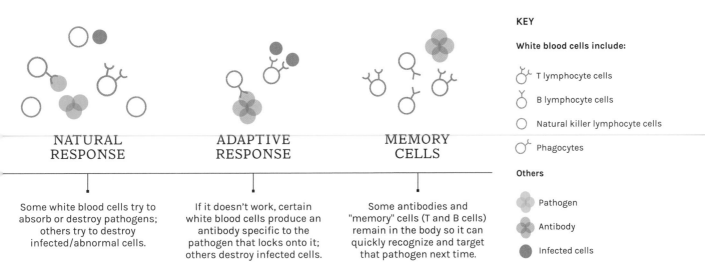

NATURAL RESPONSE

Some white blood cells try to absorb or destroy pathogens; others try to destroy infected/abnormal cells.

ADAPTIVE RESPONSE

If it doesn't work, certain white blood cells produce an antibody specific to the pathogen that locks onto it; others destroy infected cells.

MEMORY CELLS

Some antibodies and "memory" cells (T and B cells) remain in the body so it can quickly recognize and target that pathogen next time.

KEY

White blood cells include:

T lymphocyte cells

B lymphocyte cells

Natural killer lymphocyte cells

Phagocytes

Others

Pathogen

Antibody

Infected cells

SHOULD I TRY TO GET MORE VITAMIN D FROM MY DIET?

Vitamin D is essential for healthy teeth, bones, and muscle, but did you know it's technically a hormone? Unlike every other vitamin, we make vitamin D ourselves simply by the action of sunlight directly on skin, although we may need supplements.

Anyone not living at a high latitude should be able to get enough UVB light exposure to meet all their vitamin D needs in spring and summer, from about 15 minutes outside daily with legs or forearms exposed. (Cloud cover and broad spectrum sun protection may reduce exposure.) From October to March, the sun is too weak in the northern hemisphere for us to make enough vitamin D, so we need other sources to maintain our levels.

Only a few foods contain the two main forms of vitamin D: D2 (ergocalciferol) is plant based and found in fortified milks, cereals, and mushrooms. Oily fish and fish oils are good sources of D3 (cholecalciferol); one tablespoon of cod liver oil contains around 30mcg (micrograms), while other animal sources contain lower levels.

HOW MUCH DO I NEED?

Vitamin D's interaction with other nutrients enables us to build and maintain healthy bones and muscles, for example, by helping the body to absorb and conserve calcium. According to US health guidelines, most people 14-70 years old need 15mcg/600IU and people 71+ need 20mcg/800IU; since it can be difficult to obtain this much from diet, a 10mcg supplement may be necessary between October and March. People who get little or no sun exposure, those with darker skin, and children under five should consider supplementing vitamin D, based on blood lab levels. Because breast milk has low levels of vitamin D, breastfed babies and those consuming less than 17oz of formula (which is fortified) should be given an 8.5mcg supplement daily.

Vitamin D is found in many body tissues and may have multiple health impacts; a deficiency has been linked to inflammation and an increased risk of weight gain and diabetes. More positively, recent studies have identified potential benefits for female and male fertility and found that women with sufficient levels of vitamin D are less likely to miscarry.

Vitamin D3

Vitamin D from sunshine is inert and the body converts it into a biologically active form in a two-stage process.

   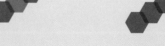

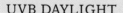

UVB DAYLIGHT	SKIN	PRE-VITAMIN D	VITAMIN D
Sun exposure UVB rays from exposure to sunlight penetrate the skin.	Enzymes in the skin UV light reacts with 7-dehydrocholesterol enzyme in skin cells.	Forming D3 Enzymes convert into pre-vitamin D, which restructures into D3.	Activating Another enzyme turns D3 into calcitriol, its active form.

Food sources of vitamin D

FOODS WITH NATURALLY SIGNIFICANT AMOUNTS OF VITAMIN D ARE SCARCE, AND PRIMARILY ANIMAL-BASED.

OILY FISH

TROUT AND SALMON ARE RICH SOURCES AT AROUND 17mcg PER 3.5oz; HERRING, MACKEREL AND SARDINES CONTAIN LESS BUT ARE STILL GOOD OPTIONS.

EGG YOLKS

EGGS FROM HENS ALLOWED TO ROAM OUTSIDE IN SUNLIGHT HAVE LEVELS OF VITAMIN D 3–4 TIMES HIGHER THAN FROM INDOOR HENS.

MEAT AND OFFAL

PORK, LAMB, BEEF, LIVER, AND KIDNEYS CONTAIN SMALL AMOUNTS OF VITAMIN D AT AROUND 0.5mcg–1mcg IN A TYPICAL PORTION.

FORTIFIED FOODS

CERTAIN FOODSTUFFS ARE FORTIFIED WITH VITAMIN D IN SOME COUNTRIES. THESE INCLUDE COW'S MILK AND SOY MILK (AND PRODUCTS MADE FROM THEM), BREAKFAST CEREALS, AND ORANGE JUICE.

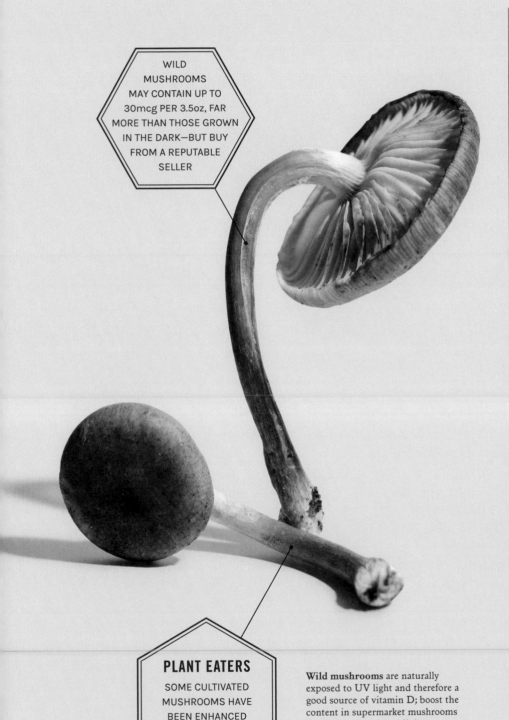

> WILD MUSHROOMS MAY CONTAIN UP TO 30mcg PER 3.5oz, FAR MORE THAN THOSE GROWN IN THE DARK—BUT BUY FROM A REPUTABLE SELLER

> **PLANT EATERS**
> SOME CULTIVATED MUSHROOMS HAVE BEEN ENHANCED WITH BIOAVAILABLE VITAMIN D

Wild mushrooms are naturally exposed to UV light and therefore a good source of vitamin D; boost the content in supermarket mushrooms by leaving them in sunlight.

DOES GUT HEALTH PLAY A ROLE IN IMMUNE RESPONSE?

While a lot remains unknown with regards to the relationship between the immune system and the gut, scientists have found some highly important links.

Research indicates that as much as 70 percent of our immune system resides in the gastrointestinal tract, including 80 percent of the body's IgA antibody-producing plasma cells. This may seem surprising until you consider that the digestive tract is the site within our bodies that receives the most day-to-day contact with external elements, mainly food and helpful gut bacteria but also pathogens and toxic substances. Not only are immune cells in the gut able to mount a defense against such harmful "foreign bodies," uniquely, they are also able to distinguish such invaders from the similarly "foreign" but needful array of nutrients in food and the microbiome of beneficial gut bacteria.

CRITICAL ROLE OF GUT BACTERIA

Scientists are also discovering how seeding of the gut microbiome helps ensure healthy development of the immune system in babies and infants. Evidence suggests gut bacteria play a key role in stimulating an expansion of intestinal immune cells; in the proper functioning of antibody secretion; and in achieving balance between the two groups of T helper cells—white blood cells that activate most other immune cells.

IMMUNE-RELATED DISORDERS

T helper cells divide into two groups: Th1 and Th2. We are born with more Th2, and bacteria colonizing the gut of newborns is needed to achieve a healthy balance between Th1 and Th2. A failure to achieve that balance, with a bias towards Th2 cells, is linked to the development of allergies. Hence some scientists theorize that poor development of infant gut bacteria could be at the root of an increasing incidence in the West of allergies and conditions that can be triggered by allergic reaction, such as asthma and eczema.

The link between allergies, autoimmune diseases, and the immune system is complex. In allergies, the immune system recognizes harmless non-invaders as harmful. In autoimmune diseases, such as celiac disease and rheumatoid arthritis, the body attacks its own tissues. There is growing evidence that composition of gut microbiota has an impact on the risk of developing these immune-related disorders.

All this need not mean your gut-immune interaction is fixed by age three. In a recent study, eating a high fiber diet that includes plenty of fermented foods (see pages 48–53), was shown to increase both the function and diversity of microbiota, leading to personalized immune responses and decreased inflammation.

Establishing your gut bacteria

Our microbiota is believed to stabilize by the age of three, remaining similar from that point into adulthood. This suggests that early life experiences may impact the composition of this bacteria, affecting us throughout our lives.

"ALT" immune systems

The immune centers of the gut are part of the lymphatic system and a wider network of lymphoid tissues that take in the nasal area, skin, and lungs—all known by acronyms ending in "ALT" for "-associated lymphoid tissue."

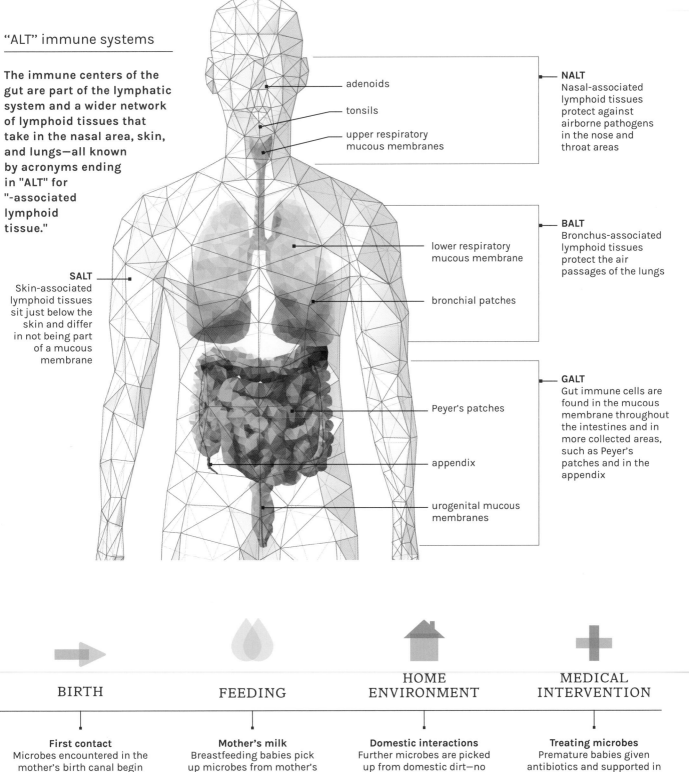

adenoids

tonsils

upper respiratory mucous membranes

NALT
Nasal-associated lymphoid tissues protect against airborne pathogens in the nose and throat areas

lower respiratory mucous membrane

bronchial patches

BALT
Bronchus-associated lymphoid tissues protect the air passages of the lungs

SALT
Skin-associated lymphoid tissues sit just below the skin and differ in not being part of a mucous membrane

Peyer's patches

appendix

urogenital mucous membranes

GALT
Gut immune cells are found in the mucous membrane throughout the intestines and in more collected areas, such as Peyer's patches and in the appendix

BIRTH

First contact
Microbes encountered in the mother's birth canal begin the process of colonizing the gut, an experience babies born by Cesarean section miss out on.

FEEDING

Mother's milk
Breastfeeding babies pick up microbes from mother's skin, and breast milk has bacteria from mother's gut as well as sugars designed to feed the microbiome.

HOME ENVIRONMENT

Domestic interactions
Further microbes are picked up from domestic dirt—no need to be overly paranoid about cleaning!—pets, and human visitors.

MEDICAL INTERVENTION

Treating microbes
Premature babies given antibiotics and supported in sterile incubators have a different mix of microbiota to full-term babies.

IS THERE A RELATIONSHIP BETWEEN SLEEP QUALITY AND NUTRITION?

It has not been fully determined whether sleep quality affects the diet and vice versa, but there does seem to be a link. What is crystal clear, however, is how important good-quality sleep is to our health and sense of well-being.

Sleep deprivation can cause health problems. During sleep, the body and mind relax and recharge, giving us energy for the next day. Much maintenance and repair work takes place in the body when we sleep.

SLEEP HYGIENE

Diet and sleep hygiene (sleep quality) seem to be linked. Having enough good-quality sleep, combined with eating regularly during the day, determines the healthy production of hormones.

Following a healthy, balanced diet (see pages 40–41) is one of the best ways of achieving good sleep hygiene. Not surprisingly, a lot of evidence links the Mediterranean diet (see pages 36–39) with better sleep hygiene and lower levels of insomnia.

POOR SLEEP HYGIENE AND WEIGHT GAIN

The relationship between insufficient sleep and obesity has been considerably researched. Insufficient sleep disrupts the hormones that govern appetite (see opposite), making us hungrier.

Research shows that people who sleep for less time often consume more calories and tend to opt for foods with a high fat content day to day than those who get sufficient sleep.

In lab experiments, sleep-deprived people tend to keep meal portions the same but snack late into the night (we've all been there!), eating on average closer to 130 percent of their daily calorie intake, with around 500 of these calories consumed late at night. At the risk of stating the obvious, from a nutritional standpoint, it makes sense to simply go to sleep when you are tired, rather than snacking to keep awake.

POOR SLEEP HYGIENE AND WEIGHT LOSS

In one study of dieters sleeping less than six hours per night, in the case of 70 percent of participants, all weight lost was from lean muscle mass, not fat. Fat is an energy-rich substance. When you don't sleep enough, cortisol levels rise, pushing the body more easily into flight-or-fight mode. The body becomes reluctant to give up fat, preferring to reserve this rich energy source for impending fight or flight. So it turns to metabolizing muscle (which is protein).

In other words, if you're trying to lose weight but getting insufficient sleep, you will lose what you want to keep—muscle—and you will hold on to what you want to lose—fat. You may be dieting diligently, managing your cravings, then unraveling all your hard work simply because of lack of sleep.

SLEEP-FRIENDLY DIETARY HABITS

Avoid foods that hinder sleep. Spicy foods, caffeine (see page 72), and alcohol can all prevent sleep.

Try a small protein/carbohydrate snack before bed. Tryptophan, an amino acid that promotes sleep, is found in small quantities in all protein foods. The best sources are eggs, soybeans, poultry, meat, fish, and cheese. It is a precursor to the sleep-inducing chemicals serotonin and melatonin. For tryptophan to have a sedative effect, it needs to be consumed with a carbohydrate food.

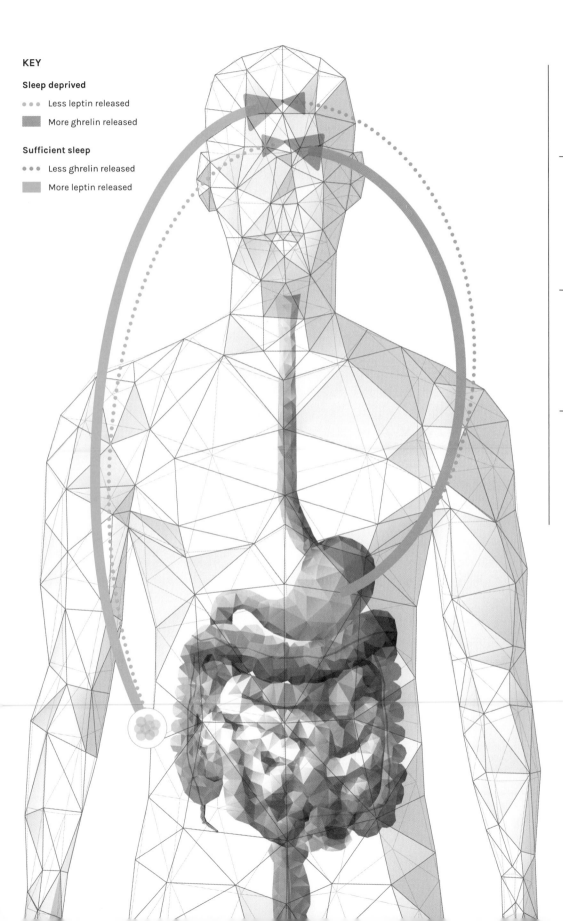

KEY

Sleep deprived

••• Less leptin released

▪ More ghrelin released

Sufficient sleep

••• Less ghrelin released

▪ More leptin released

7–9 hr
SLEEP PER
NIGHT IS
RECOMMENDED

7% OF
AMERICANS GET

9+ hr
SLEEP
PER NIGHT

60% OF
AMERICANS GET

7–8 hr
PER NIGHT

33% OF AMERICANS
GET ONLY

6 hr
OR FEWER
PER NIGHT

Sleep deprivation
causes disruption of many
hormones, including those
that govern sleep (see page
105). More ghrelin (the
hunger hormone) than
normal is released when
sleep deprived, while less
leptin (the satiety hormone)
is present, leading to
snacking and overeating.
This is reversed when
you've had enough sleep.

CAN DIET HELP REDUCE MENSTRUAL SYMPTOMS?

Half of the world's population experiences menstruation during their lifetimes, yet there has not been much good-quality research exploring how diet influences menstruation and period pain.

What we know is that certain nutrients (see opposite) seem to reduce symptoms, so it makes sense to try to include them in your diet daily.

PMS

Premenstrual syndrome (PMS) is a combination of physical and psychological complaints experienced during the days leading up to menstruation and once bleeding begins. Symptoms include low mood and mood swings, headache, bloating, lower backache, breast tenderness, acne, and fatigue.

An estimated 30–40 percent of women experience PMS, with 77 percent experiencing psychological symptoms and 71 percent suffering from tiredness and, in some cases, debilitating exhaustion. One in three women report being unable to perform as usual.

Low calcium and vitamin D levels may exacerbate symptoms. Research shows that supplementing and/ or consuming foods rich in these nutrients may help relieve symptoms. Take a 10mcg supplement of vitamin D. Iron may help increase energy levels. As the body loses iron in menstrual blood, it makes sense to ensure dietary sources of iron are kept high during menstruation to avoid risk of a deficiency.

CRAMPS

Dysmenorrhea (cramps) is the most common period symptom, affecting 85 percent of women. When menstruation begins, there is a rise in inflammatory compounds called prostaglandins. These cause the uterine muscle to contract and release blood.

Magnesium and omega-3 may help relieve the cramping sensation by reducing contractions. Recent studies show that supplementation with omega-3 fatty acids, known for their anti-inflammatory properties, may reduce pain intensity. Similar results are shown with fish oils.

Supplementation with vitamins D and E and ginger may also reduce the severity of cramps. Ginger contains gingerol and gingerdione, which may have anti-inflammatory and analgesic effects.

There is some limited evidence indicating that a low-fat vegetarian diet and calcium supplements reduce the duration and intensity of period pains.

DIGESTIVE COMPLAINTS

Many people report digestive discomfort and a change in bowel habits during their period, with the most disruption occurring on day one. In the days leading up to this day, levels of the hormones estrogen and progesterone rise in preparation for a possible pregnancy. These hormones are known to slow gastrointestinal motility.

Focus on eating as well as possible, including lots of fiber in the diet and drinking plenty of water to keep bowel movements healthy. It also makes sense to reduce your consumption of foods that can increase inflammation of the gastrointestinal tract and cause bloating, such as alcohol, caffeine, fatty foods, and fizzy drinks. Some (uncontrolled) research suggests that habitual caffeine intake is associated with menstrual abnormalities.

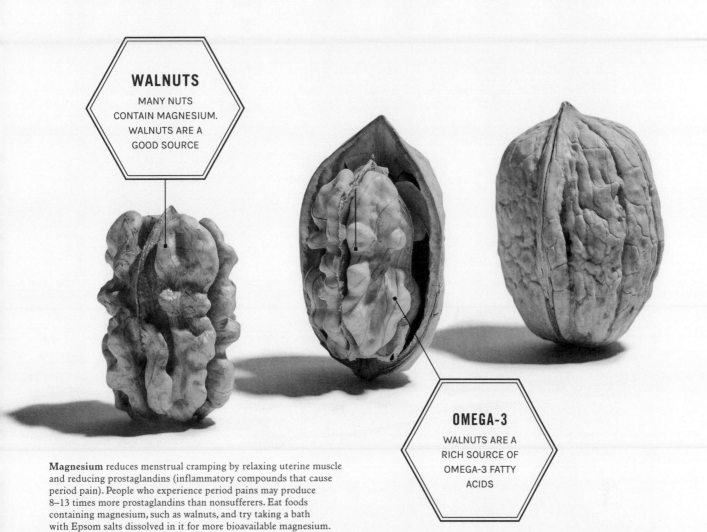

WALNUTS
MANY NUTS CONTAIN MAGNESIUM. WALNUTS ARE A GOOD SOURCE

OMEGA-3
WALNUTS ARE A RICH SOURCE OF OMEGA-3 FATTY ACIDS

Magnesium reduces menstrual cramping by relaxing uterine muscle and reducing prostaglandins (inflammatory compounds that cause period pain). People who experience period pains may produce 8–13 times more prostaglandins than nonsufferers. Eat foods containing magnesium, such as walnuts, and try taking a bath with Epsom salts dissolved in it for more bioavailable magnesium.

SOURCES OF

MAGNESIUM	OMEGA-3	CALCIUM	VITAMIN D	IRON
PUMPKIN SEEDS	SALMON	MILK	SALMON	LIVER
WALNUTS	TROUT	CHEESE	MACKEREL	RED MEAT
BRAZIL NUTS	MACKEREL	YOGURT	HERRING	LEGUMES
ALMONDS	SARDINES	FORTIFIED MILKS	SARDINES	NUTS
CASHEW NUTS	FLAXSEEDS	FORTIFIED BREAD	RED MEAT	EGGS
PEANUTS	CHIA SEEDS	SARDINES WITH BONES	EGG YOLKS	DRIED FRUITS
SUNFLOWER SEEDS	CANOLA OIL	CANNED SALMON WITH BONES	FORTIFIED FOODS	POULTRY
SOYBEANS	AVOCADOS	KALE	MUSHROOMS EXPOSED TO SUNLIGHT	FISH
WHEAT-BASED FOODS	SOYBEANS	ORANGE		WHOLE GRAINS
COOKED SPINACH	LEAFY VEGETABLES	BROCCOLI		DARK LEAFY GREENS
	WALNUTS			

SHOULD I EAT DIFFERENTLY FOR MENOPAUSE?

The symptoms of menopause still aren't discussed openly enough, even though half of the population will experience them to varying degrees—all the more reason to talk about whether certain foods could help ease this major life transition.

For most women, menopause is a natural aging process during which they lose their period due to declining estrogen levels. Plant compounds called phytoestrogens may help ease hot flashes and night sweats, the most common symptoms. So far, research has focused on one type—isoflavones—found in soybeans and soy-based foods and drinks. Only 10%–20% of Asian women experience hot flashes compared with a large majority of perimenopausal or menopausal women in the US, where soy intake is lower.

Findings from research into soy's impact on symptoms have been mixed. However, a 2021 review of more than 400 studies concluded that eating around 50mg (milligrams) of isoflavones daily is associated with both reduced frequency and severity of hot flashes. This amount can be obtained from two servings of soy foods or drinks within a balanced diet. Scientists don't yet understand the precise mechanism, but isoflavones appear to produce a weak estrogen-like effect without actually affecting estrogen levels.

Soy-based cheese and meat alternatives often have added salt and more fat than tofu, tempeh, and soybeans, so eat these less often. Caffeine and alcohol can also exacerbate hot flashes.

BREAST CANCER RISK

Some breast cancers are estrogen-dependent, and studies have identified a link between soy and increased risk. The 2021 review concluded that isoflavones are chemically different to estrogen, and soy isoflavones are safe to eat as part of a healthy diet without increased risk of breast cancer occurring or recurring. This is based on eating up to 100mg of isoflavones daily—around 9oz of tofu

Does soy always help?

Soy isoflavones have a similar, though not identical, chemical structure to human estrogen, which means they can act in different ways to ostrogen. Some people may experience mild estrogen-like effects, like less severe hot flashes, and others no effects.

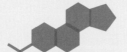

HUMAN ESTROGEN

Human estrogen is able to bind to a similar degree to both types of estrogen receptors found on organs and tissues around the body.

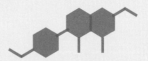

SOY ISOFLAVONE

Soy isoflavones prefer to bind to one type of estrogen receptor and may affect the body differently to human estrogen, such as having an antioxidant effect.

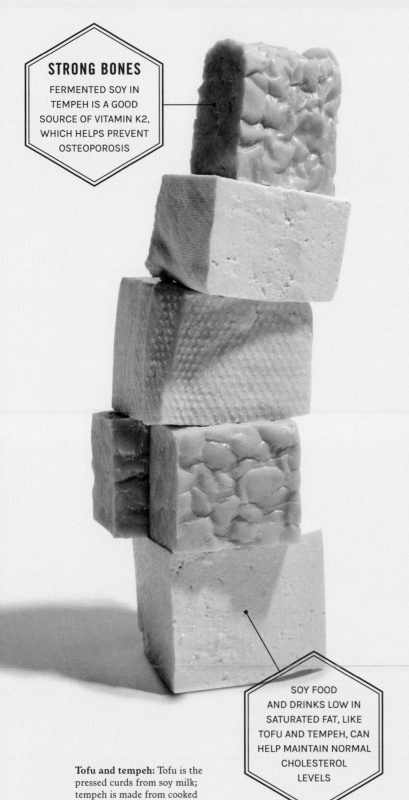

STRONG BONES

FERMENTED SOY IN TEMPEH IS A GOOD SOURCE OF VITAMIN K2, WHICH HELPS PREVENT OSTEOPOROSIS

SOY FOOD AND DRINKS LOW IN SATURATED FAT, LIKE TOFU AND TEMPEH, CAN HELP MAINTAIN NORMAL CHOLESTEROL LEVELS

Tofu and tempeh: Tofu is the pressed curds from soy milk; tempeh is made from cooked soybeans and is fermented.

or up to 29oz of soy milk. (It may still be best to take medical advice before consuming high-dose phytoestrogen supplements.)

HEART AND BONE HEALTH

Postmenopausal women are at a higher risk of cardiovascular disease and should eat less salt and more fiber and replace saturated fats with unsaturated. Calcium is also important because menopause can accelerate the age-related decline in bone mineral density. You should get a sufficient amount in a healthy diet from sources, including leafy greens, calcium-fortified foods, dairy products, and fish eaten with bones. It's also crucial to get enough vitamin D alongside calcium, and supplements may be required, especially if suffering from osteopenia and osteoporosis (see pages 138–139).

DAILY SOY BOOST

TWO SERVINGS OF SOY-BASED FOODS MAY HELP ALLEVIATE HOT FLASHES AND IS BROADLY EQUIVALENT TO:

3.5oz REGULAR CUBED TOFU
HALF BLOCK (3.5oz) TEMPEH
3.5oz EDAMAME BEANS
2 x 8.5oz SOY MILK
1 x 8.5oz SOY MILK + 7oz PLAIN SOY YOGURT ALTERNATIVE

CAN I EAT TO SUPPORT THE AGING PROCESS?

As well as affecting appearance, flexibility, and cognitive health, getting older may increase our chances of developing a noncommunicable disease. Can diet help us live longer and improve well-being in later years?

———

By 2050, there are expected to be two billion people over 60, more than double the number in 2015. Aging increases the risk of developing chronic conditions like type 2 diabetes, cancer, or heart disease, but scientists don't yet fully understand the complex mechanisms behind it. One theory says antioxidants obtained from diet (like vitamins C and E, selenium, and zinc) may help protect us from potentially harmful free radical molecules and the damage to cells that speeds up as we age. Research indicates that it's safer to obtain these nutrients

from a balanced diet, including a wide range of plants, rather than from supplements; these often contain highly concentrated doses the body may not require, and too many could have damaging effects.

MEDITERRANEAN EATING

Evidence generally points to a correlation between healthy lifestyle and lower risk of chronic disease. One study based on long-term data found that those who routinely ate a Mediterranean-style diet with plenty of vegetables, whole grains, and fish were 30

How excess sugar ages skin

———

Collagen and elastin keep skin firm but can be damaged by glycation. This process is accelerated by eating a lot of high GI (glycemic index) food, especially sugary foods, that rapidly convert to sugar in the blood.

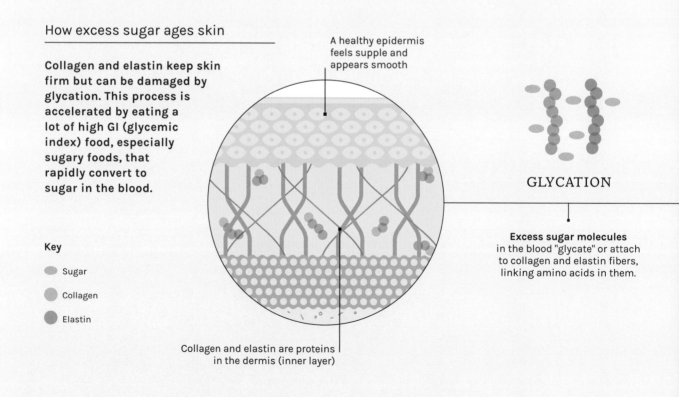

A healthy epidermis feels supple and appears smooth

GLYCATION

Excess sugar molecules
in the blood "glycate" or attach to collagen and elastin fibers, linking amino acids in them.

Key

- Sugar
- Collagen
- Elastin

Collagen and elastin are proteins in the dermis (inner layer)

percent more likely to age successfully (defined as reaching 70 with no major mobility problems or chronic disease, no loss of cognitive skills, and good psychological health). Researchers tracking data on nearly half a million middle-aged adults found an overall healthy lifestyle, including diet, could increase male life expectancy by 6 years and female life expectancy by 7.5 years.

SKIN AGING

After age 20, collagen production gradually declines, and the number and size of skin cells reduces, making skin thinner. Fatty fish like salmon and mackerel may help support skin cells. Antioxidants in fruits and vegetables—especially vitamins A (beta carotene), E and C, lycopene, and lutein—may neutralize harm done by free radicals. Broaden your intake and include kale, carrots, spinach, red peppers, tomatoes, and turnip greens. Adults may also want to eat 2–3

Brazil nuts daily for skin-supporting selenium; researchers have found that two 2oz servings of almonds daily for six months led to significantly less severe wrinkles.

JOINT AND BRAIN SUPPORT

As we age, we lose muscle mass and bone density, increasing the risk of osteoporosis and frailty. Between ages 19–70, healthy adults should aim to consume 1,000mg of calcium for men and 1,200mg for women a day to protect bone health and enough vitamin D to absorb it (see pages 138–139). Older people (and breastfeeding women) should get at least 1,200mg. To help muscles repair and grow, aim to eat a portion (about palm size) of protein at each meal, such as chicken breast, beans and lentils, and tofu. Doing some weight-bearing exercise is important, too. Several studies have also found an association between lower overall mental decline and eating unsaturated fats (see pages 150–151).

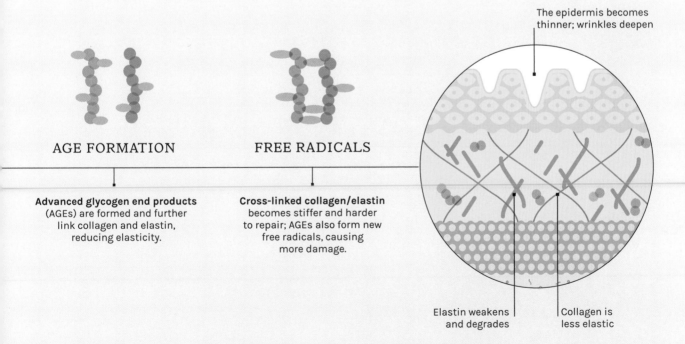

AGE FORMATION

FREE RADICALS

The epidermis becomes thinner; wrinkles deepen

Advanced glycogen end products (AGEs) are formed and further link collagen and elastin, reducing elasticity.

Cross-linked collagen/elastin becomes stiffer and harder to repair; AGEs also form new free radicals, causing more damage.

Elastin weakens and degrades

Collagen is less elastic

CAN I EAT TO GUARD AGAINST DEMENTIA?

"Dementia" describes different cognitive impairments that are often minor to start with, then become severe enough to affect daily life. Adopting healthy eating habits before reaching later years may be one way to reduce your risk.

Dementia symptoms include difficulties with problem-solving or communication, loss of memory, and mood swings. There are many kinds of dementia, and specific symptoms depend on the underlying cause. In Alzheimer's disease, the leading cause, structural changes in the brain cause cells to die, while restricted blood supply can cause vascular dementia. When it develops in older age, in some cases, dementia is thought to be lifestyle related.

DEMENTIA AND DIET

Evidence indicates a healthy weight and lifestyle in midlife lessen the chances of developing dementia. A body of research also shows a positive association between cognition and diet; while this doesn't establish causation, it points toward eating a varied, Mediterranean-style diet low in salt, sugar, and saturated fat and rich in vegetables and whole grains. Refined carbohydrates, including sugars added to many processed foods, are absorbed quickly and prompt a bigger insulin response than complex carbohydrates. People with type 2 diabetes appear to be at higher risk of dementia, but research into the reasons why is still at an early stage. It's possible that excess insulin enables a protein called beta-amyloid to accumulate faster in the brain.

BRAIN FOOD?

Scientists designed the MIND (Mediterranean-DASH Intervention for Neurogenerative Delay) diet to combine elements of two other diets that studies show are both beneficial for reducing the risk of type 2 diabetes and cardiovascular problems.

Notably, though, it emphasizes leafy greens (although eating other vegetables is important) and berries, because their antioxidant properties can help reduce oxidative stress, an imbalance between free radicals and protective antioxidants in the body that can lead to cell damage.

Otherwise, some studies indicate eating more omega-3 fatty acids reduces the chance of developing dementia; good sources include oily fish (see pages 42–43). However, others found no effects, so longer-term research is needed. A high level of compounds called advanced glycation end products (AGEs) is associated with the inflammation and oxidative stress that precede many chronic diseases, including Alzheimer's; these may also contribute to the tangling of Tau proteins inside brain cells. AGEs form inside the body when blood glucose combines with proteins or fats; high levels may also form in foods exposed to high-temperature cooking.

AGE LEVELS AND COOKING

BEEF HIGH	**BEEF** LOW
FRIED | 9,522	STEWED | 2,443
CHICKEN HIGH	**CHICKEN** LOW
ROASTED | 5,975	BOILED | 2,232
SALMON HIGH	**SALMON** LOW
GRILLED | 3,012	POACHED | 2,063
POTATOES HIGH	**POTATOES** LOW
FRIED | 694	BOILED | 17

Alzheimer's and the brain

Billions of neuron cells transmit information around the brain,
then to the body. Alzheimer's interferes with their communication and
repair processes and causes greater loss of neurons than normal.
Scientists are still investigating exactly why this happens.

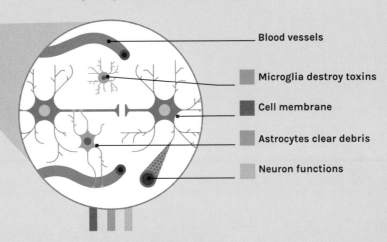

HEALTHY BRAIN

NETWORKS OF NEURONS
COMMUNICATE VIA ELECTRICAL AND
CHEMICAL (NEUROTRANSMITTER)
SIGNALS ACROSS GAPS CALLED
SYNAPSES AND CONTINUALLY
REPAIR THEMSELVES.

Blood vessels

Microglia destroy toxins

Cell membrane

Astrocytes clear debris

Neuron functions

WHEN THINGS GO WRONG

BETA-AMYLOID

IN ALZHEIMER'S BRAINS,
AN ABNORMAL AMOUNT OF
THIS NORMALLY HARMLESS
WASTE PRODUCT COLLECTS
BETWEEN NEURONS
AND FORMS
PLAQUES

"SUPPORT" CELLS

INSTEAD OF REMOVING DEBRIS
LIKE BETA-AMYLOID, MICROGLIA
AND ASTROCYTE CELLS
CAUSE INFLAMMATION
AND FURTHER DAMAGE
NEURONS

TAU PROTEINS

NORMALLY, THESE
SUPPORT NEURONS'
INTERNAL STRUCTURE; IN
ALZHEIMER'S, THEY FORM
TANGLES THAT DISRUPT
NEURONS' SIGNALING
FUNCTION

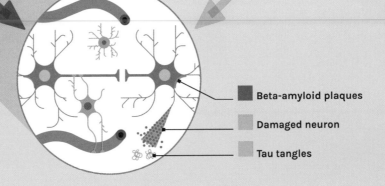

ALZHEIMER'S BRAIN

AS MORE NEURONS ARE DAMAGED AND
DIE, COMMUNICATION BETWEEN
NETWORKS BREAKS DOWN AND AREAS
OF THE BRAIN SHRINK. AT FIRST, THIS
AFFECTS MEMORY: LATER, LANGUAGE,
REASONING, AND BEHAVIOR.

Beta-amyloid plaques

Damaged neuron

Tau tangles

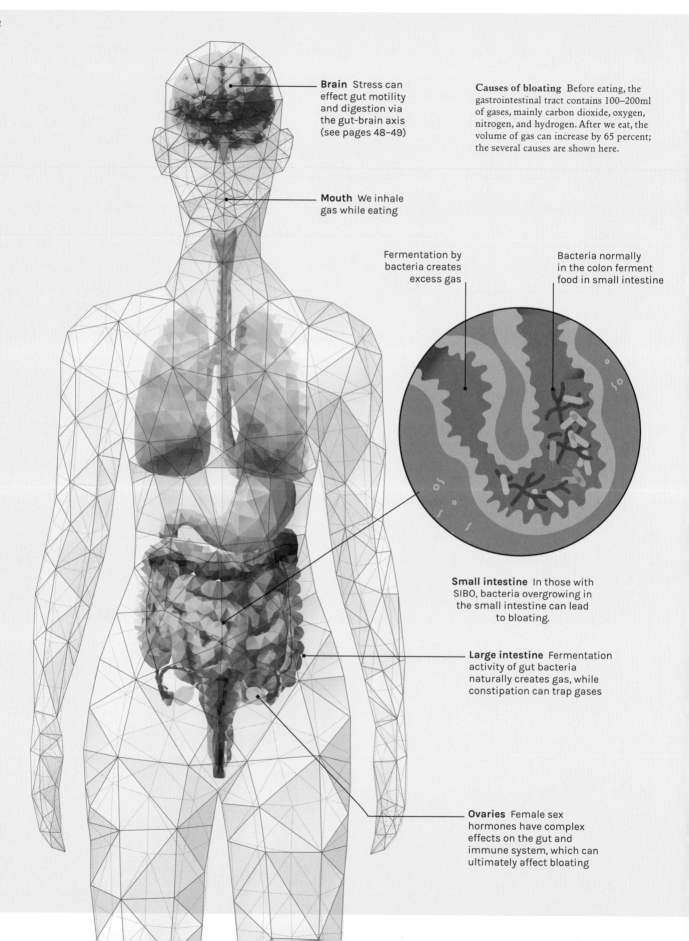

Brain Stress can effect gut motility and digestion via the gut-brain axis (see pages 48–49)

Causes of bloating Before eating, the gastrointestinal tract contains 100–200ml of gases, mainly carbon dioxide, oxygen, nitrogen, and hydrogen. After we eat, the volume of gas can increase by 65 percent; the several causes are shown here.

Mouth We inhale gas while eating

Fermentation by bacteria creates excess gas

Bacteria normally in the colon ferment food in small intestine

Small intestine In those with SIBO, bacteria overgrowing in the small intestine can lead to bloating.

Large intestine Fermentation activity of gut bacteria naturally creates gas, while constipation can trap gases

Ovaries Female sex hormones have complex effects on the gut and immune system, which can ultimately affect bloating

WHY DO I FEEL BLOATED?

Bloating is the sensation associated with gas in our gut, when your abdomen feels swollen and is commonly distended. It can make us feel uncomfortably full and is sometimes accompanied by pain, flatulence, and nausea.

Even in a "fasted" state, our gastrointestinal tract contains gases, which increase after eating due to swallowing air and gases produced during digestion. But it is normal for our stomachs to distend when we eat a meal—they are not supposed to remain flat!

Eating high-fiber foods, such as legumes, may lead to bloating due to increased gas production in the large intestine; but for many, fiber can reduce bloating by improving digestion and speeding up gut transit. When we swallow, air enters our stomach and can lead to abdominal distention. This is enhanced when we eat too quickly or drink a lot of liquid while eating, especially carbonated drinks. Other key contributing factors include:

Stress Feeling stressed can affect communication mechanisms of the gut-brain axis (see pages 48–49), for example, by changing levels of neurotransmitters, which can disturb our ability to digest foods well and lead to constipation or diarrhea by affecting gut motility.

Hormones Women report feeling bloated more than men, probably due to differences in sex hormones and fluctuations in their levels. Progesterone rise before a period can promote bloating and other digestive issues; whereas estrogen stimulates gut muscle relaxation by inducing nitric oxide synthase.

Gut microbiota Our gut bacteria breaks down indigestible foods, producing gases as a by-product. More bloating is experienced in those with IBS (see page 164) due to visceral hypersensitivity. Studies have shown that the amount of gas produced is actually similar to healthy individuals.

Constipation Delay in passing stool and increase in stool bulk leads to the accumulation and trapping of gases, exacerbated by the longer time spent in the large bowel, which increases bacterial fermentation.

Small intestine bacterial overgrowth (SIBO) Most gut bacteria live in our large intestine. SIBO occurs when these grow in the small intestine and disrupt digestion and absorption, leading to bloating.

Sensitive gut Evidence has emerged for a condition called visceral hypersensitivity, which describes greater sensitivity or perception to bloating and other symptoms. Patients with gastrointestinal disorders are particularly prone to sensitive gut.

Intolerances For those with food intolerances, eating such foods can lead to bloating. For example, the lactose intolerant do not have the enzyme to digest lactose in cows' milk, so this is broken down by gut bacteria instead, producing excess gas.

Can you treat it?

THERE IS NO ONE-SIZE-FITS-ALL CURE, AND TREATMENT PLANS TEND TO BE PERSONALIZED. They range from lifestyle changes relating to diet, exercise, and stress; to administering probiotics; to medications such as laxatives in those with constipation or antibiotics for SIBO sufferers. Identifying the potential cause is important for addressing underlying conditions, for example, dietary issues in patients with IBS or food intolerances. While bloating is common and fairly normal, do see your primary care physician if this is persistent to rule out any gastrointestinal disorders.

IS IT NORMAL TO FART?

Flatulence might feel embarrassing, but it is perfectly normal to pass wind and an important part of digestion. You will never hear a nutritionist shying away from discussing farts!

Most people fart 5 to 15 times a day. Farting is a sign of a healthy gut microbiome (see pages 48–49), but if it becomes foul smelling or increases in frequency, it may need investigating.

EXCESS GAS

We fart because of natural fermentation in the gut. There can be several reasons for producing abnormal quantities of gas: feeding the gut too much; when we can't digest certain foods because of a food intolerance; if you suddenly increase the amount of fiber in the diet, this can shock the body as it isn't used to working that hard; or if food travels too quickly through our intestines, for example, when we get diarrhea. Conversely, if food moves too slowly through our intestines and we become constipated, the fermentation process has a long time to "brew" food that would have normally been excreted, producing gas as a by-product.

UNPLEASANT ODORS

Mostly, the gas we produce when we pass wind has no odor. Foul-smelling farts happen when our gut breaks down sulfur-containing compounds, which contributes to sulfur-containing—and smelly—gases like hydrogen sulfide. If you experience these smells frequently, it may be worth looking at your diet and speaking to a registered dietitian nutritionist for some help.

Red cabbage Not only cabbage, but all vegetables in the Brassica family cause smelly farts.

Foods that can contribute to sulfurous wind include:
- **Animal proteins**—meat, protein powders, eggs
- **Plant foods**—broccoli, cabbage, cauliflower, garlic, onions
- **Drinks**—wine, beer

While everyone is unique, many scientists report high protein intake as the main cause of smelly wind, and advise action to lower levels of protein in the diet first (see page 15 for recommended intakes), before cutting back on any plant foods. By safely and slowly increasing fiber in the diet from plant-based foods, you may actually help gut microbiota by enabling them to break down food at a consistent pace instead of waiting around in a stop-start manner.

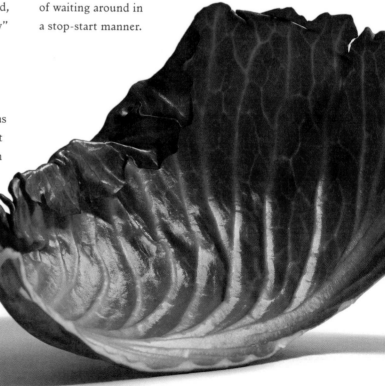

WHY AM I CONSTIPATED?

Constipation can be frustrating and sometimes painful, resulting in a lot of straining and hard poop.

Food that can't be digested by your body goes into your large intestine, where it mixes with fluid to form poop. Bowel muscles then tense and relax to push poop toward your bottom. If you often find it difficult to poop, you may be constipated:

- **Slow transit constipation** occurs when your stool takes such a long time to get through the large intestine, much of its water content is absorbed and it turns hard and dry.
- **Evacuation disorder** comes down to the final push to excrete the stool, when coordination of the muscles involved is poor. This could have been a result of childhood toilet habits or be a structural problem of your biology.
- **Constipation-predominant irritable bowel syndrome** is a type of IBS mostly owed to constipation (see page 164).

CONSTIPATION IN CHILDREN

Our digestive system undergoes changes from birth to adulthood, but especially in the first year of life with the introduction of solids, and constipation is a common symptom of weaning. Children with abdominal pain often simply have constipation but should always be checked out.

HOW CAN I RELIEVE CONSTIPATION?

Drink a minimum of 6–8 cups water per day and gradually increase fiber in your diet from plant foods. Fiber provides bulk to poop since it isn't absorbed through the gut lining; fiber also absorbs water, softening poop. Exercise can also help with gut motility. Laxatives are helpful in some situations, for example, post-childbirth and in those with a lot of pain, but they can also make constipation worse and you may become dependent on them, which can influence gut microbiota and toilet habits. Sitting on the toilet with your back straight at 90 degrees to your legs can cause the intestine to be pinched. Adopt a more "crouching" position with your legs at 35 degrees to your torso; a foot rest can be helpful.

CABBAGE

GLUCOSINOLATES ARE SULFUR-CONTAINING PHYTOCHEMICALS IN CABBAGE THAT CAN CAUSE ODOROUS FARTS

SIGNS OF CONSTIPATION INCLUDE

POOPING LESS THAN THREE TIMES A WEEK

DIFFICULTY AND PAIN WHEN POOPING

STRAINING A LOT WHEN POOPING

POOP LIKE SMALL HARD PELLETS

A FEELING YOU HAVEN'T BEEN ABLE TO GET ALL THE POOP OUT

IS DIARRHEA CAUSED BY DIET?

Diarrhea is a condition where you pass loose, watery stools more frequently than is normal and can be triggered by a whole host of things from stress to travel, anxiety, and the food we eat.

Each day, nine liters of water enter our small intestine, 90 percent of which is reabsorbed. Diarrhea occurs when there is too much water in the intestine or not enough of it is reabsorbed. While diarrhea causes dehydration, simply drinking more water can make severe diarrhea worse and may require an oral rehydration solution instead.

ELECTROLYTE LOSS

A bout of diarrhea can leave you with an imbalance of electrolytes—minerals, including sodium, potassium, and calcium, that help regulate fluids in the body and facilitate proper functioning of cells. Replenish electrolytes with rehydration powders or by drinking milk or coconut water. Short-term diarrhea can be managed at home for most people, but chronic diarrhea can be a cause for concern, so visit your primary care physician as soon as possible.

CONTAMINATED FOOD AND WATER

Diet may cause diarrhea when bacteria, such as *Campylobacter* or *Escherichia coli* (*E. coli*), enter the body through contaminated food; or a parasite, such as that which causes giardiasis (contributing to gastritis), enters in contaminated water. These are common causes of diarrhea when vacationing in places with poor hygiene standards: practice good hygiene (see right) and avoid potentially unsafe tap water and undercooked food.

FOOD TRIGGERS

If you have a food intolerance, this can lead to loose stools; and diet may also trigger IBS symptoms, which can include diarrhea (see pages 158–167).

Other more general food-related causes include:
- **Spicy food** can irritate the stomach lining.
- **Fatty fried foods** contain saturated fats and trans fats, which the body can sometimes struggle to break down, leading to diarrhea or worsening symptoms.
- **Coffee** stimulates your digestive system, as well as making you mentally alert, and many people have a bowel movement soon after a cup of coffee.
- **Drinking alcohol** can lead to loose stools the next day, especially when drinking beer or wine.
- **High FODMAP foods** containing Fermentable, Oligosaccharides, Disaccharides, Monosaccharides and Polyols can cause diarrhea. For example, garlic and onions contain fructans, which is a carbohydrate some people with IBS find difficult to digest. (They also contain insoluble fiber, which can make foods move through the digestive system faster.)
- **Some artificial sweeteners** can upset the digestive system, so much so that foods containing them may have labels warning of their laxative effect.

Good hygiene

REDUCE YOUR RISK OF DEVELOPING DIARRHEA FROM CONTAMINANTS BY MAINTAINING HIGH STANDARDS OF HYGIENE:

Wash your hands thoroughly with soap and warm water after going to the bathroom and before eating or preparing food.

Clean the toilet, including the handle and the seat, with disinfectant after each bout of diarrhea.

Avoid sharing towels, sheets, or utensils with other household members.

Food poisoning

E. coli bacteria are naturally present in the intestines of humans and animals and help with digestion, but certain toxin-producing strains ingested through contaminated food and water can cause diarrhea.

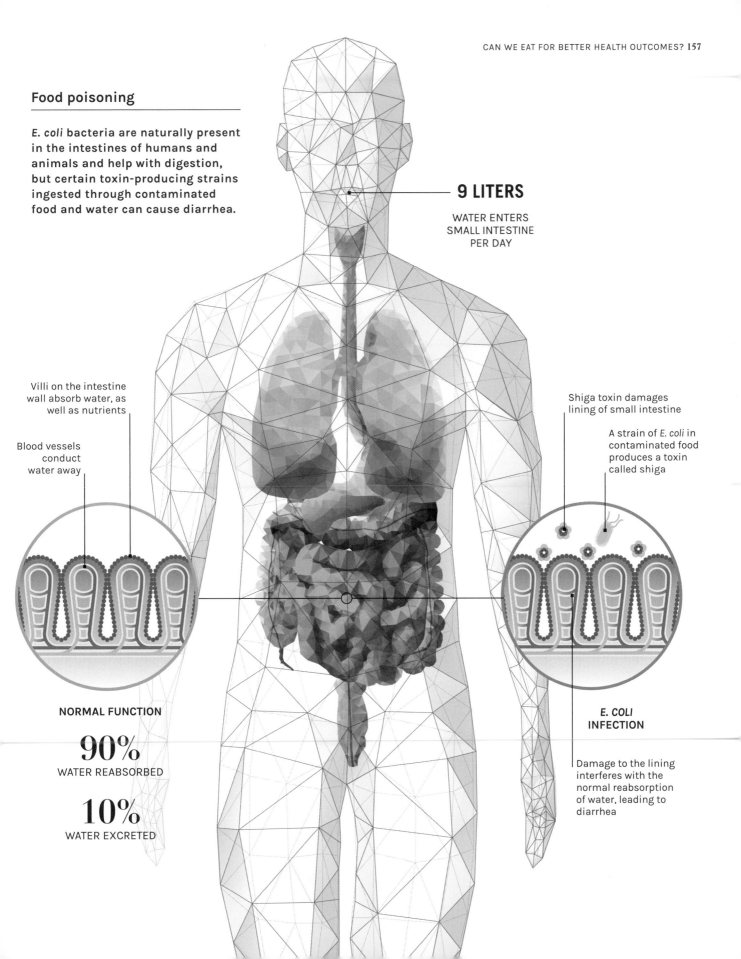

9 LITERS
WATER ENTERS
SMALL INTESTINE
PER DAY

Villi on the intestine wall absorb water, as well as nutrients

Blood vessels conduct water away

Shiga toxin damages lining of small intestine

A strain of *E. coli* in contaminated food produces a toxin called shiga

NORMAL FUNCTION

90%
WATER REABSORBED

10%
WATER EXCRETED

E. COLI
INFECTION

Damage to the lining interferes with the normal reabsorption of water, leading to diarrhea

SHOULD I BE WORRIED ABOUT FOOD ALLERGIES AND INTOLERANCES?

Abnormal responses to eating food, or "adverse food reactions," can be the result of either a food intolerance (often called sensitivity) or a food allergy. Despite often being lumped together, these are two very different reactions.

All of us experience digestive discomfort from time to time; if mild and infrequent, there is usually no cause for concern. However, regular discomfort after eating may indicate an allergy or intolerance. Allergies can be severe and in some cases life threatening, so it's important to know the signs. About 2 percent of adults and 4–8 percent of kids in the US have a food allergy; intolerances seem more prevalent.

FOOD ALLERGIES

A food allergy is an adverse immune response. It usually comes on suddenly and can be triggered by a small amount of food. The allergic reaction will occur every time you consume the food, regardless of how much you eat or how frequently you eat it. There are two different types of allergic responses. IgE-mediated allergies are when the body creates antibodies specific to the food that has been digested. These allergies can be lifelong, with symptoms ranging from hives and swelling to anaphylactic shock. Non-IgE-mediated food allergies involve other components of the immune system. These reactions come on more slowly and are harder to diagnose, with symptoms including bloating, vomiting, and diarrhea.

Several factors can cause food allergies, including diet, environment, and genetics. The dual-allergen exposure hypothesis suggests that early exposure to

IgE-mediated allergic reaction

When IgE first binds an allergen to a dendritic cell, it starts a process to produce more allergen-specific IgEs. The IgEs then stick to mast cells (an immune cell) in the digestive tract, ready to react to the same protein when it is consumed again.

KEY

- white blood cell—T cells
- white blood cell—B cells
- IGE (immunoglobulin E)
- allergen
- Inflammatory (histamine)

dendritric cell

IGE

DENDRITIC CELL AND ALLERGEN

The body creates immunoglobulin E (IgE) antibodies specific to a protein in the allergen food

IgE binds an allergen to a dendritic cell, sending a message to T cells

food allergens via the skin (for instance, nut oils in moisturizers) could increase the likelihood of allergy, while consumption of those allergens in infancy could encourage tolerance. Researchers have linked early and regular consumption of peanuts to prevention of peanut allergy, particularly in children at higher risk because of a compromised skin barrier, such as those with eczema. (Whole nuts and peanuts should not be given to children under five due to choking risk.)

INTOLERANCES

An intolerance is a nonimmune response that directly impacts digestion. Intolerances often relate to the amount of food consumed or the frequency of consumption. Some are triggered by certain chemicals in food, while others develop if you lack the enzymes needed to break down a specific food. While not life threatening, food intolerances can greatly impact quality of life. Symptoms tend to come on gradually and can include rashes, itching, bloating, and diarrhea (the last two can also be caused by other diseases, such as bowel cancer, so get them checked out by your doctor).

THE DIET-INDUSTRY TRAP

It may seem like everyone has an intolerance these days, with seemingly more and more people changing their diets for fear of food intolerance. But there is no evidence to account for the rise; the apparent increase is more likely due to self-reporting and fad diets than actual incidences. One study found that 34 percent of parents reported food allergies in their children but only 5 percent were found to have an allergy.

The media is rife with misinformation that encourages people to waste money on expensive products they don't need. Unregulated alternative health therapists are diagnosing people with intolerances they don't have, potentially delaying a correct diagnosis from a qualified health professional (see pages 160–161). Excluding common staples, such as bread, from our diets can even lead to malnutrition. What's more, a developing concern is that by restricting foods unnecessarily, people may become more at risk of developing an eating disorder. See a credentialed health professional for a proper diagnosis or advice, and make changes to your diet according to their guidelines.

FOODS THAT PEOPLE CAN BE INTOLERANT TO INCLUDE:

LACTOSE

MILK AND OTHER LACTOSE-CONTAINING PRODUCTS

MANY TABLETS HAVE LACTOSE ADDED AS A FILLER

VASO-ACTIVE AMINES

RED WINE, STRONG AND BLUE CHEESES, TUNA, MACKEREL, PORK PRODUCTS, AND OTHER FOODS

NATURAL CHEMICALS

SUCH AS SALICYLATE AND GLUTAMATE

SOME FOOD ADDITIVES

ESPECIALLY BENZOATE, SULFITE PRESERVATIVES, AND MONOSODIUM GLUTAMATE

See more on common triggers on pages 160–161

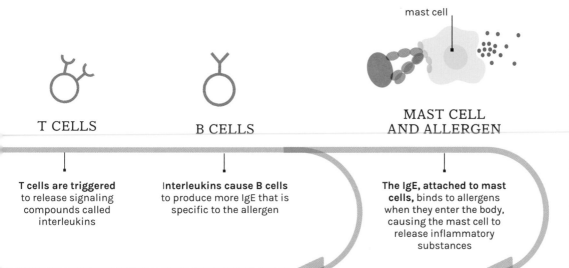

T CELLS

B CELLS

MAST CELL AND ALLERGEN

mast cell

T cells are triggered to release signaling compounds called interleukins

Interleukins cause B cells to produce more IgE that is specific to the allergen

The IgE, attached to mast cells, binds to allergens when they enter the body, causing the mast cell to release inflammatory substances

HOW CAN I FIND OUT IF I HAVE AN ALLERGY OR INTOLERANCE?

Food allergies and intolerances can make life very difficult, so if you think you have one, it's important to ask for medical support in identifying, treating, and managing the issue.

Figuring out whether you suffer from an allergy or intolerance can be a difficult process. There are many unanswered questions in the scientific world about allergies. If you are worried, it's best to seek help from a doctor before eliminating a food group completely, to enable you to get tested correctly and avoid any nutritional deficiencies. It's a good idea to keep a food diary and monitor your symptoms.

DIAGNOSING FOOD ALLERGIES

There are many foods that people can be allergic to, some of the most common being milk, wheat, eggs, peanuts, tree nuts, fish, shellfish, and some fruits and vegetables. In addition, some food additives can increase the symptoms of an existing allergy.

For instance, sulfites, used to preserve food, can cause some people with asthma to have an attack, though it is not necessary for all asthma sufferers to avoid them. Oral allergy syndrome is a less common type of allergy, in which the body mistakes the protein in some fruits or vegetables for pollen, causing symptoms such as an itchy mouth and/or throat, and mild swelling in the mouth area.

Celiac disease (where the small intestine is hypersensitive to gluten) is technically not a food allergy, but an autoimmune disease caused by an allergic reaction to gluten, a group of proteins found in wheat, barley, and rye. It is thought to affect at least 1% of Americans; however, only about 30 percent of people with the condition are currently

Lactose intolerance

Lactose is a type of sugar found in most dairy products. In humans, the enzyme lactase is needed to break down lactose, so when the body doesn't produce enough lactase, the lactose passes through the gut undigested, leading to symptoms of intolerance, such as cramps and bloating.

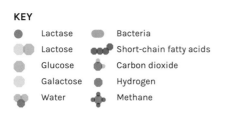

KEY

● Lactase	● Bacteria
◑ Lactose	●●● Short-chain fatty acids
● Glucose	● Carbon dioxide
● Galactose	● Hydrogen
● Water	✚ Methane

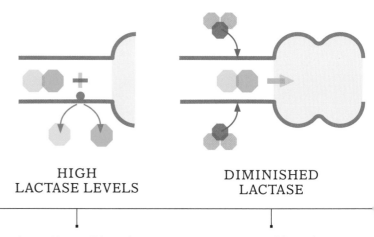

HIGH LACTASE LEVELS

Digested in small intestine
Lactase splits lactose into glucose and galactose, which can be absorbed into the blood

DIMINISHED LACTASE

Passes small intestine
Undigested lactose moves to the large intestine and causes increased water in the colon

clinically diagnosed. Symptoms may include cramps, bloating, nausea, and reflux. It is possible to have a wheat allergy and not have celiac disease, or to have nonceliac gluten-sensitivity (though little is known about this).

Not much is known about why people develop allergies. If someone in your family has or had an allergy, you will be more likely to develop one, too, though not necessarily the same one. Those with allergies often have other conditions, such as asthma and hay fever.

An IgE-mediated food allergy (see pages 158–159) can be diagnosed either by measuring the antibodies present in the blood or by inserting allergens into the skin and looking for a reaction. Alternatively, a supervised elimination diet can help you figure out what the allergen is.

SPOTTING FOOD INTOLERANCES

The list of foods that can cause digestive discomfort is long. Common triggers include food additives such as MSG, caffeine, alcohol, artificial sweeteners and preservatives, a group of carbohydrates known as FODMAPs (see pages 166–167), eggs, yeast, fructose, and even toxins that enter food. Few food intolerances are lifelong, and in most cases, people can eat small amounts without enduring problems.

Two of the most widely discussed food intolerances are to wheat and lactose. Gluten is often mistakenly blamed for digestive discomfort, but gluten intolerances are not medically recognized, and a lot of the time the symptoms may be due to something else, such as IBS, stress, anxiety, IBD, or celiac disease. Lactose is a disaccharide sugar mainly found in dairy products. An intolerance occurs when a person lacks the enzyme lactase (see below) so cannot break down the disaccharide into monosaccharides glucose and galactose to then enter the blood. This can lead to a buildup of lactose in the digestive system, resulting in wind, cramps, diarrhea, bloating, and nausea. (See pages 162–163 for more on cutting gluten and lactose from your diet.)

There is currently no clinically valid test for diagnosing an intolerance. Instead, they are confirmed by cutting out suspected trigger foods and observing symptoms, followed by gradual reintroduction of the excluded foods.

ALLERGIES

MILK

PEANUTS

TREE NUTS

FISH

SHELLFISH

SOME FRUITS AND VEGETABLES

SOY

CELERY

MUSTARD

SESAME

PINE NUTS

MEAT

EGGS WHEAT

INTOLERANCES

MSG

CAFFEINE

ALCOHOL

ARTIFICIAL SWEETENERS

ARTIFICIAL FOOD PRESERVATIVES

FODMAPS (see pp.166–167)

YEAST

FRUCTOSE

LACTOSE

GLUTEN

VASO-ACTIVE AMINES (found in red wine, strong and blue cheeses, tuna, mackerel, pork products, and other foods)

SALICYLATES

Allergies and intolerances Some foods can cause allergies while others may cause intolerances. Some foods may cause both.

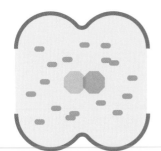

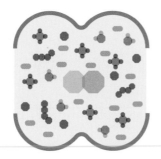

FERMENTATION   BY-PRODUCTS

Digestion in colon
The lactose is digested by gut bacteria instead, causing fermentation

Cramps and bloating
The increase in acids and gas caused by fermentation can lead to cramps and bloating

HOW DO I CUT GLUTEN OR LACTOSE FROM MY DIET?

If you've been told by your doctor to eliminate either gluten or lactose from your diet, it may seem like a daunting prospect, but you can do so successfully without compromising on nutrition.

GLUTEN SOURCES

GLUTEN CAN BE FOUND IN ALL SORTS OF PRODUCTS, IN FOODS YOU MIGHT NOT EXPECT

FLOUR

BREADS AND OTHER BAKED GOODS

CEREALS

PASTA

COOKIES

CAKES

SOY SAUCE

BEER

SOUPS

PROCESSED MEATS

READY-MADE SAUCES

READY MEALS

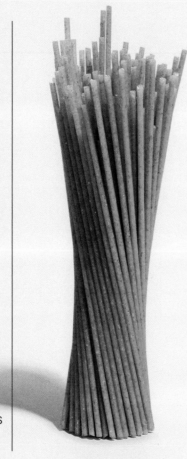

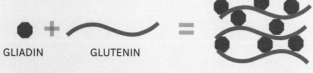

GLIADIN + GLUTENIN = GLUTEN

What is gluten? The proteins gliadin and glutenin combine with water to create a mesh structure known as gluten, which has an elastic quality that is especially useful in baking.

The majority of people won't need to cut gluten or lactose from their diets, but those who are advised to often see dramatic benefits to their health and energy levels, provided they maintain a healthy, balanced diet with alternative foods. Consult a doctor or registered dietitian to figure out what exactly you need to exclude, and remember that while going gluten-free can have positive outcomes for some, for others it may do more harm than good.

ELIMINATING WHEAT OR GLUTEN

Be aware of the difference between wheat and gluten if you need to avoid one or both. If diagnosed with celiac disease (when the immune system reacts abnormally to gluten), you may need to exclude rye, barley, and oats from your diet as well as gluten. Some individuals with a wheat allergy (which occurs when the body produces antibodies to proteins found in wheat) will be able to have a variety of grains, and others will not; for most, it is safest to eliminate gluten entirely. Gluten-free products are not always wheat-free and vice versa, so check labels.

Gluten is found in many everyday products (see left). It also crops up in convenience foods, so be sure to check labels carefully. Thankfully, it's possible to buy wheat-free or gluten-free versions of these food items. In addition to flour, baking powder can also be wheat- or gluten-free. And watch out for xanthan gum, which is often added to baking items to help with the texture and binding of the mixture; those who have celiac disease or gluten intolerance often react to this, too.

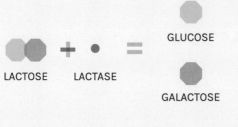

GLUCOSE

LACTOSE LACTASE

GALACTOSE

Lactose digestion Lactose is a natural sugar found in milk. It is broken down in the small intestine by the enzyme lactase into two simple sugars, glucose and galactose, which are then absorbed into the blood.

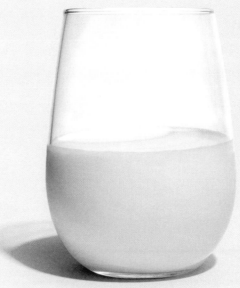

Gluten-free products are lower in fiber and often higher in fat and sugar than their gluten-containing equivalents, and since they are not governed by the same fortification rules as wheat products, they may also contain fewer vitamins and minerals, including iron, B vitamins, and calcium. Gluten-free products are also lower in protein given that the gluten (protein) is removed.

ELIMINATING LACTOSE

Like the gluten/wheat distinction, there is a difference between lactose intolerance and a milk allergy. The former results from a lack of lactase, the enzyme that breaks down lactose into more easily absorbed sugars (see above and pages 160–161). The latter is an immune reaction to one of the many proteins in animal milk, though it's most often caused by the alpha S1-casein protein in cow's milk. Bear in mind that while lactose-free products don't contain the sugar lactose, they may still contain milk proteins.

When eliminating lactose-containing foods, think about the vitamins and minerals you would be getting in the original product and aim to replace them elsewhere in your diet. Look for foods that contain calcium, vitamins D and B12, and iodine, in particular. For instance, B12 and iodine are found in fish and eggs. Lactose-free products contain the same vitamins and minerals as standard dairy products, but they also have lactase added, which helps the body digest any lactose taken in. Rice, oat, almond, cashew, quinoa, soy, and pea milk are all great dairy-free milk alternatives (though rice milk should not be given to under-fives due to its arsenic content).

Cow's milk is often added to manufactured foods, so it isn't just a simple case of eliminating obvious dairy products, such as milk, butter, cheese, and yogurt. For common ingredients derived from cow's milk, see right.

BEING MINDFUL

You will need to be vigilant about everything you eat, to avoid cross-contamination. In the US, it's law that allergens must be clearly mentioned on food packaging, usually emphasized in bold and listed in one place. "May contain" statements are often used on packaging to state that a food may be contaminated with one or more common allergens. Restaurants and cafés must also provide all dietary information on allergens in writing and communicate them verbally.

LACTOSE SOURCES

LACTOSE CAN BE FOUND IN NUMEROUS MILK PRODUCTS, PROTEINS, AND INGREDIENTS

BUTTERMILK

CALCIUM OR SODIUM CASEINATE

CASEIN (CURDS), CASEINATES

COTTAGE CHEESE

GHEE

HYDROLYZED CASEIN

HYDROLYZED WHEY PROTEIN

LACTOALBUMIN

LACTOGLOBULIN

LACTOSE

MARGARINE

MILK PROTEIN

MILK SOLIDS

MILK SUGAR

MODIFIED MILK

WHEY AND WHEY SOLIDS

COULD I HAVE IRRITABLE BOWEL SYNDROME (IBS)?

If you suffer from digestive discomfort and don't believe it to be caused by a food intolerance, it's possible you could have IBS—though see a doctor to be sure.

Irritable bowel syndrome is the most common type of functional gastrointestinal disease, with global prevalence ranging from 2–15 percent. IBS is more common in women, and, unlike many illnesses, incidence decreases with age. Symptoms vary and can change over time, but commonly include bloating, constipation, and/or diarrhea, and recurrent abdominal pain—to be diagnosed with IBS, you must have experienced frequent abdominal pain for at least three months, with symptom onset at least six months prior to diagnosis.

DIAGNOSIS AND TREATMENT

The mechanisms behind IBS are still unclear, but research suggests that they are multifactorial and patient dependent. IBS is now considered a disorder of the gut-brain axis (see page 49); in many cases, it can be caused by stress. Certain molecules in food may play a large part, too (see page 166). Since IBS mimics other disorders, it is often hard to diagnose.

Doctors tend to start by assessing a patient's clinical history to identify and rule out other diseases, then perform a physical examination, sometimes requiring laboratory tests and colonoscopies. There are four IBS subtypes: IBS-C (constipation predominant), IBS-D (diarrhea predominant), IBS-M (mixed bowel habits), and IBS-U (unclassified).

Not everyone responds to IBS treatments in the same way. Often, changes to diet and lifestyle are recommended first; then you may try antibiotics, antispasmodics, antidepressants (as neuromodulators that can impact gut motility, visceral hypersensitivity, and gastrointestinal transit speed), laxatives, or antidiarrheal drugs, as well as cognitive behavioral therapy (CBT) and other psychological interventions. However, the treatments are by no means a cure and tend to target only one part of what is a multi-modal condition. Reducing or eliminating intake of certain foods can be effective (see pages 166–167).

Intestinal spasms
A common symptom of IBS, intestinal spasms occur when the muscles of the gut contract spontaneously, causing irregular bowel movements and abdominal pain.

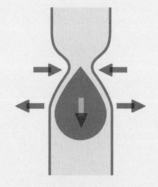

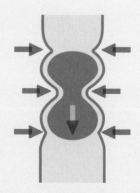

NORMAL SEQUENCE

SPASM

WHAT IS IBD?

Often confused with IBS, irritable bowel disease (IBD) refers to two conditions causing inflammation of the gastrointestinal tract: Crohn's disease and ulcerative colitis.

Crohn's disease can affect any part of the gastrointestinal (GI) tract, from the mouth to the anus, though in most patients, the lower part of the small intestine is affected. Inflammation is patchy and can extend through multiple layers of the GI tract walls. In ulcerative colitis, the inflammation is confined to the colon (or large intestine) and rectum. This condition causes ulcers to develop on the inner lining of the bowel, which may bleed and produce mucus. Symptoms of both types of IBD include persistent diarrhea, abdominal pain, rectal bleeding, weight loss, and fatigue.

As with IBS, the causes of IBD are not yet fully understood. Researchers believe that diet, stress, immunity, and genetics are all factors, with risk levels dependent on age, ethnicity, family history, cigarette smoking, and high usage of nonsteroidal anti-inflammatory drugs (NSAIDs).

IBD is diagnosed first through testing levels of fecal calprotectin, then with an endoscopy or colonoscopy and biopsies. There are a number of medications that can be used in treatment, but diet can also play a huge role, especially in those with mild IBD. Doctors also recommend that IBD patients are given a number of vaccinations to prevent infections. In severe cases, a patient may undergo surgery to remove damaged portions of the GI tract, though this has become less common thanks to advances in treatment with medications.

Celiac disease

WHILE NOT A FORM OF IBD ITSELF, CELIAC DISEASE CAN CAUSE SIMILAR SYMPTOMS. The condition causes your immune system to attack your own tissues when you eat gluten, damaging the small intestine's lining, which can decrease absorption of nutrients. If untreated, complications can include anemia, osteoporosis, infertility, neurological conditions and nerve damage, and, rarely, small bowel cancer and intestinal lymphoma. (See also page 160.)

Inflammation patterns
While both sorts of IBD feature inflammation, the location of it differs between Crohn's and UC.

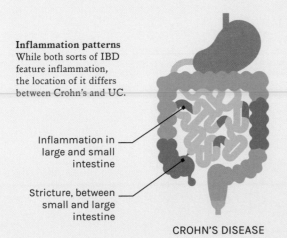

Inflammation in large and small intestine

Stricture, between small and large intestine

CROHN'S DISEASE

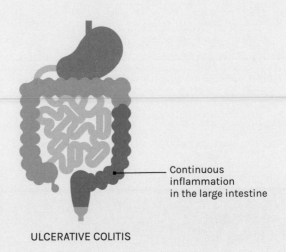

Continuous inflammation in the large intestine

ULCERATIVE COLITIS

WHAT ARE FODMAPs AND CAN AVOIDING THEM CURE IBS?

If you have made changes to your lifestyle to improve symptoms of Irritable Bowel Syndrome (IBS; see page 164) but had no results, the next approach may well be to work with a registered dietitian nutritionist on what is known as the low-FODMAP diet.

FODMAPs—fermentable, oligosaccharides, disaccharides, monosaccharides, and polyols—are a group of carbohydrates that the small intestine cannot digest. When we eat them, they pass through to the large intestine where they are fermented by gut bacteria. Many foods fall into the FODMAP category, including apples, avocados, pears, mangoes, cauliflower, soybeans, rye, beans, and pulses.

"Fermentable" covers foods that can be fermented and used as food for gut bacteria. Oligosaccharides are a type of carbohydrate that usually contains 3–10 simple sugar molecules, such as fructans, found in onions, garlic, wheat, rye, and barley, and galacto-oligosaccharides (GOS), found in beans and lentils.

Disaccharides, such as lactose, contain two simple sugar molecules, and monosaccharides, such as fructose, contain one sugar molecule. Polyols, also known as "sugar alcohols," are sorbitol and mannitol, which are mainly found in sugar-free sweets, mints, and chewing gum, plus certain fruits and vegetables.

HOW FODMAPS CAUSE SYMPTOMS

The mechanisms behind FODMAP symptom production are not fully known, but there are two main hypotheses:

● The "small bowel hypothesis" states that FODMAPs are osmotically active molecules (i.e., triggering the diffusion of water from an area of high concentration

Stomach

Small intestine

Large intestine

FODMAPs in the gut

FODMAPs may trigger excess water to either form in the small intestine or ferment in the large intestine, causing gut discomfort.

FOODS HIGH IN FODMAPs

Garlic, onions, broccoli, cauliflower, mushrooms, apples, pears, watermelon, cherries, and wheat products such as pasta and pastries are all classed as FODMAP foods

to an area of low concentration through a selectively permeable membrane), which cause an increase in water in the small intestine, leading to distension, bloating, and discomfort.

● The "large bowel hypothesis" suggests that FODMAPs increase colonic bacterial fermentation as well as gas production. This results in bloating, flatulence, and discomfort. It is also thought that psychological factors and an altered brain–gut axis (see p.49) caused by stress, anxiety, and a hectic lifestyle may play a role.

THE LOW-FODMAP DIET

The low-FODMAP diet (LFD) is a popular and effective way to ease IBS symptoms and improve patient quality of life. In fact, it has been proven to reduce gut symptoms in patients with IBS 70–80 percent of the time. While it can seem highly restrictive, if followed correctly, this diet allows for individual personalization. It is incredibly important to embark upon the LFD only with supervision, to ensure you remain healthy throughout. Patients have two or three appointments with a dietary specialist, and there are three stages in the process:

1. Elimination: A period of four to six weeks when patients must restrict all FODMAPs from their diet. At the end of this period, they should see symptom improvement.

2. Reintroduction: Over the following weeks, patients begin to reintroduce FODMAPs into their diet systematically, adding one food at a time back into the diet in increasing quantities, allowing the patient to identify their symptom threshold for each of the FODMAPs.

3. Personalization: Over time, patients can personalize their diet, adding in the FODMAPs that don't cause symptoms and reducing or eliminating those that do, to control symptoms while maintaining a nutritionally adequate diet.

If you think you have IBS, speak to your GP. While the LFD has excellent results in some people, only follow it if advised to do so and with professional support. It's also not recommended to stay on the diet for a long period of time, as reduced gut microbiome diversity, which can be a result of the LFD, can be more detrimental to gut health in the long term.

FODMAPs

ARE A GROUP OF INDIGESTIBLE CARBOHYDRATES FERMENTED IN THE LARGE INTESTINE

F
FERMENTABLE

O
OLIGOSACCHARIDES

D
DISACCHARIDES

M
MONOSACCHARIDES

A
AND

P
POLYOLS

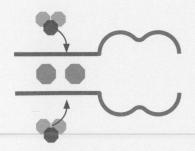

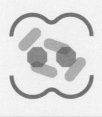

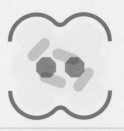

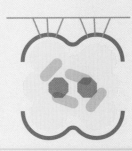

SMALL INTESTINE	BACTERIAL REACTION IN LARGE INTESTINE	GAS BUILDS UP = EXPANSION	MESSAGE SENT TO NERVOUS SYSTEM
If the reaction takes place in the small intestine, then water is absorbed via osmosis, leading to distension and bloating	Bacteria in the large intestine react with the food eaten to cause fermentation	The muscle wall expands with the build up of gas as a result of the fermentation	The large intestine sends a signal via the expanded muscle to the nervous system

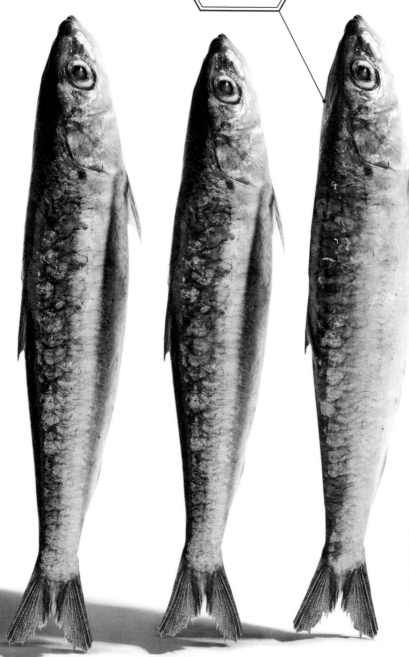

SARDINES

PROVIDE PROTEIN, CALCIUM, AND VITAMINS B12 AND D AS WELL AS OMEGA-3 FATTY ACIDS

Sources of omega-3 Fish such as sardines, mackerel, herring, salmon, and snapper have a darker flesh that is rich in omega-3 fatty acids. Vegan DHA supplements are also an option.

WHAT IS AN
ANTI-INFLAMMATORY DIET?

There isn't such a thing as an anti-inflammatory diet, but there may be a link between diet and inflammation. This area needs more research, but there's no harm in trying a few recommendations to see how they work for you.

Inflammation is a natural process, the body's normal response to some types of injury or illness (cuts or colds, for instance). It is part of your body's defense system and the process of healing.

In some cases, people have chronic inflammation in the body. Arthritis, asthma, eczema, some heart and lung diseases, diabetes, and some cancers all involve chronic inflammation. The gut is susceptible to inflammation in some. Chronic inflammatory conditions of the gut include IBS and IBDs such as celiac disease (see pages 164–165).

DIETARY CAUSES OF INFLAMMATION

Many studies have looked into the potential link between the food we consume and inflammation. These show that consuming the following foods and beverages in excess may cause inflammation:

- refined carbohydrates, such as white bread, cakes, and pastries
- French fries and other fried foods
- soda and other sugar-sweetened beverages
- red meat (like burgers or steaks) and processed meats (like hot dogs or sausage)
- margarine, shortening, and lard

Try limiting these items in your diet if you experience inflammation regularly.

REDUCING INFLAMMATION

Inflammation is a response of the immune system, and gut health has been linked to good immunity (see pages 140–141). This may be how we are able to have some influence on our immune health. Aim for a good diet that supports your gut microbiota.

Certainly, a healthy diet is unlikely to aggravate inflammation, but there is no conclusive evidence linking specific foods to reducing inflammation, except in the case of rheumatoid arthritis (RA).

In one study, one group of people with RA was given a diet rich in fiber, oily fish, and probiotics, while another was provided one of protein, red meat, and saturated fat. Members of the first group experienced a health improvement. We need more research to explore these findings, but following dietary recommendations for people with RA (increase omega-3s, calcium, and iron) may reduce inflammation in other parts of the body. Some research shows a reduction of RA symptoms if following a Mediterranean diet (see pages 36–39).

Omega-3 fatty acids

PEOPLE WITH RHEUMATOID ARTHRITIS ARE ADVISED TO INCLUDE OMEGA-3 IN THE DIET.
Fish oils have been shown to help dampen general inflammation and may help reduce joint pain and stiffness. Try to eat two 5oz (140g) portions of oily fish per week. Some eggs and breads are enriched with omega-3. Omega-3 fats from plant sources (such as flaxseed, evening primrose, and borage oil) have a weaker effect on reducing inflammation and are of limited benefit. High-dose fish oil supplements (500–1000mg of EPA and DHA per capsule) have been shown to reduce symptoms of RA. Be patient—it can take up to three months for symptom relief. Speak to your doctor before taking any new supplements.

WHAT IS DIABETES AND WHAT ARE THE RISK FACTORS?

Diabetes is a condition in which you have elevated levels of glucose in your blood. Type 1 diabetes, an autoimmune disease, has sudden onset and is not caused by diet. The onset of type 2 is gradual and less severe and is heavily influenced by diet.

When glucose is obtained from diet, it is released into the bloodstream for the body to use as fuel (see pages 12–13). The hormone insulin, supplied by the pancreas, helps cells access this fuel. People with diabetes have a problem with insulin, which means their cells cannot access glucose for fuel. Glucose remains in the bloodstream, causing hyperglycemia (high blood glucose levels). Sustained hyperglycemia can damage the eyes, kidneys, and heart.

In people with type 1 diabetes, the pancreas is unable to make insulin. The absence of insulin makes it impossible for the body to access glucose for energy, forcing it to break down fat instead. This releases fatty acids called ketones into the body. These can make the blood acidic, resulting in a life-threatening complication known as diabetic ketoacidosis (DKA).

In people with type 2, the pancreas fails to supply enough insulin. To gain more energy, the body signals to the pancreas to release more insulin. The pancreas then works very hard to pump out insulin, resulting in such high levels of insulin in the blood that cells become less sensitive to it (insulin resistance). The pancreas also becomes damaged.

TYPE 1

NO INSULIN PRESENT
GLUCOSE LEVELS RISE, CAUSING HYPERGLYCEMIA OR, IN SOME CASES, DKA.

TYPE 2

LOW INSULIN LEVELS
CAUSING HYPERGLYCEMIA. MORE INSULIN IS RELEASED, DAMAGING THE PANCREAS OVER TIME

Insulin enables cells to access glucose

Insulin "unlocks" the cells, enabling glucose to enter so the cell can use it as a source of energy. When a person has diabetes, this system can break down at various stages.

Small intestine

Pancreas

Insulin

GLUCOSE BECOMES AVAILABLE

INSULIN IS RELEASED

Glucose is released
from carbohydrates that are broken down in the small intestine. It enters the bloodstream

In response to a rise
in blood glucose levels, the pancreas produces and releases the hormone insulin

KEY

⬡ Glucose

⬡ Insulin

RISK FACTORS

Approximately 8 percent of people with diabetes have type 1 and 90 percent have type 2. There may be a genetic risk involved in developing type 1 diabetes. With type 2, there is a strong genetic risk factor—the child of a parent with type 2 has roughly a one-in-three chance of developing it. The more distant the genetic relationship, the slimmer the chance of developing the condition.

Ethnicity is also a factor: South Asian, Chinese, Black African, and African Caribbean people have a higher chance of developing type 2 than people of other ethnicities.

Age is important. People over 40 (or younger in ethnic groups more at risk) are at higher risk.

Being overweight or obese also increases the risk of developing type 2 diabetes, especially if you carry excess body fat around the abdomen.

DIET AND DIABETES

Type 1 is a lifelong condition for which insulin injections and consistent medical monitoring are necessary. No dietary interventions can prevent or reverse it, although diet plays a role in managing the condition.

Hyperglycemia symptoms

IF YOU EXPERIENCE THESE SYMPTOMS, ASK YOUR DOCTOR FOR A BLOOD SUGAR CHECK:

- extreme thirst (polydipsia)
- frequent urination (polyuria)
- physical exhaustion
- weight loss and loss of muscle mass
- genital thrush (frequent, minor infections)
- slow healing of cuts and wounds
- blurred vision.

When it comes to type 2 diabetes, the number of people being diagnosed is growing at a shocking rate. This is a health crisis in the making and, to a large degree, it is preventable. It's important that people with a risk factor are aware that there is much they can do to avoid developing the condition (see pages 172–173). The same advice can help those who have already been diagnosed with type 2 diabetes to improve their symptoms and even reverse the condition.

TYPE 2

INSULIN RESISTANCE CELLS RESPOND LESS TO INSULIN. GLUCOSE IS UNABLE TO ENTER THE CELL, CAUSING HYPERGLYCEMIA

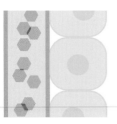

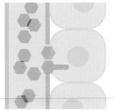

INSULIN AND GLUCOSE LEVELS RISE

Insulin and glucose are now in the bloodstream in relatively appropriate quantities, ready for the body's cells to use

INSULIN OPENS CELL

Insulin binds to a cell wall and effectively opens the cell, like a key in a lock, to allow glucose to enter the cell

GLUCOSE ENTERS CELLS

Glucose enters the cell and is used for energy in the cell respiration process, or turned into glycogen (see page 30) to be stored for later use

CAN DIET HELP PREVENT OR MANAGE TYPE 2 DIABETES?

Yes! A healthy diet in conjunction with regular exercise and weight management drastically reduces the chances of developing type 2 diabetes and can help manage—and even reverse—the condition if it has already developed.

You are at a high risk of developing type 2 diabetes (prediabetes) if your blood sugar levels are consistently high and you experience symptoms of hyperglycemia (see page 170). While not everyone with prediabetes goes on to develop diabetes, a high percentage do.

Certain dietary choices can help prevent type 2 diabetes if you are prediabetic, but diet alone will not do it. You need a healthy lifestyle overall. People with a genetic risk factor (see page 171) with more sedentary lives are more likely to develop type 2 diabetes than those who exercise regularly.

The same dietary choices can help "reverse" type 2 diabetes. This term is used to describe a significant long-term improvement in insulin sensitivity (see page 170) in people with type 2 diabetes. Those who can get their HbA1c below 42 mmol/mol (6 percent) without taking diabetes medication are said to have reversed or resolved their diabetes or brought it into remission. (This is not the same as completely eliminating it, as unwise dietary and lifestyle choices could reestablish the condition, and permanent damage to the pancreas may also have been done.)

DIETARY MEASURES

There's no one-size-fits-all approach to getting your diet right, but the previous advice to avoid sugar altogether and cut carbs is no longer recommended. People with prediabetes or type 2 diabetes should enjoy all the food groups and a balanced healthy diet, like the Mediterranean diet (see pages 36–39). Include plenty of fiber (see pages 18–19) and opt for whole grains to help keep blood glucose levels steady. Even small changes can make a difference, such as consuming whole fruit rather than fruit juice.

Portion control, to avoid overeating, is important for preventing and controlling type 2 diabetes. Mindful eating (see pages 206–207) can help make you stop eating on autopilot and become more aware of your eating patterns. Take a moment to assess how you feel before you reach for a food item. Are you doing so out of habit, or boredom, or are you actually

TESTING BLOOD SUGAR LEVELS

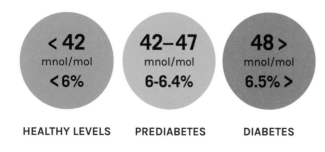

< 42 mnol/mol <6%	42–47 mnol/mol 6-6.4%	48 > mnol/mol 6.5% >
HEALTHY LEVELS	PREDIABETES	DIABETES

To diagnose diabetes, levels of gylcated hemoglobin (Hb1Ac) are tested over a period of 2–3 months. When the body is unable to use glucose properly (see pages 170–171), unused glucose in the bloodstream sticks to red blood cells (hemoglobin)—they become glycated. High Hb1Ac levels indicates prediabetes or diabetes. As blood cells are renewed every 2–3 months, testing across this period reveals an average reading.

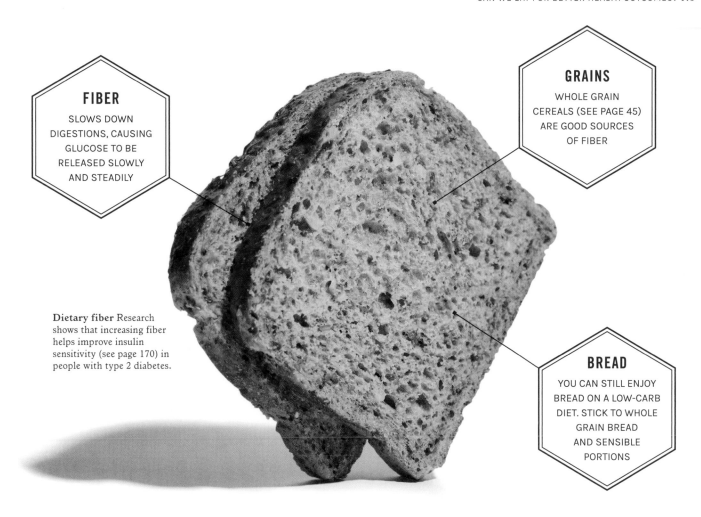

FIBER

SLOWS DOWN
DIGESTIONS, CAUSING
GLUCOSE TO BE
RELEASED SLOWLY
AND STEADILY

GRAINS

WHOLE GRAIN
CEREALS (SEE PAGE 45)
ARE GOOD SOURCES
OF FIBER

Dietary fiber Research
shows that increasing fiber
helps improve insulin
sensitivity (see page 170) in
people with type 2 diabetes.

BREAD

YOU CAN STILL ENJOY
BREAD ON A LOW-CARB
DIET. STICK TO WHOLE
GRAIN BREAD
AND SENSIBLE
PORTIONS

thirsty rather than hungry? Questions like
these can help you identify unhelpful habits.

LOW-CARB DIET

One of the few cases in which a low-carb diet
is recommended is in the case of type 2 diabetes.
Research indicates that following a low-carb
diet is an effective way to reverse the condition.
A trial showed that consuming 50–130g carbs
per day helped manage weight and improve
blood sugar levels and cardiovascular risk in
people with type 2 diabetes who were tested
for up to 12 months.

If you have type 2 diabetes and are considering
a low-carb diet, get the support of a dietitian to
ensure your diet is nutritionally adequate. When

a macronutrient is removed from the diet in
this way, the knock-on effects can be dangerous
(see pages 110–111). For instance, carbs contain
fiber, which helps control blood sugar levels and
keeps the gut microbiome happy (see pages
48–53). Suddenly reducing carbs can result in
constipation (see page 155). More research is
needed to identify the best dietary patterns on
a low-carb diet to maintain normal blood sugar
levels and keep fiber intake up.

If you are on certain meds (including insulin
or gliclazide), there is a possible risk with a
low-carb diet of hypoglycemia or, in rare cases,
ketoacidosis (see page 170). Speak to your doctor
to help you manage risks and adjust medication
as necessary.

30g

**FIBER
PER DAY**

HELPS KEEP
BLOOD
GLUCOSE
STEADY

EXAMPLES:

WHOLE GRAINS
LEGUMES
FRUITS
NUTS
SEEDS
VEGETABLES

DO SOME FOODS CAUSE OR PREVENT CANCER?

Despite what you might have read on the internet, no one food or dietary pattern directly causes—or cures—cancer, so there's no need to be overly restrictive with your diet. Food is not medicine, but it is essential to overall health and happiness.

Good nutrition during and beyond cancer treatment can help maintain a healthy weight, retain muscle mass and strength, and decrease overall side effects. If you have cancer, please speak to your doctor or dietitian before changing diet; the internet is full of dangerous advice, and it is best to seek support from credentialed health professionals to be safe.

CANCER FOOD MYTHS
Here are some of the top food myths around cancer that you should be extremely wary of:

● **Acidic foods** You may have read that eliminating acidic foods and eating only alkaline foods can cure cancer. The "alkaline diet" is based on a notion that the food we eat has the potential to change how acid or alkaline our blood is, but this is scientifically not true (see opposite). Our bodies are tightly regulated,

and lungs and kidneys maintain blood pH behind the scenes. There is no link at all between eating acidic foods and cancer.

● **Juicing** Associated with the alkaline diet myth is a belief that consuming juices derived from alkaline ingredients can purge the body of acid and so cure cancer. Not only is this treatment highly unethical, it is incredibly dangerous and can be life threatening (see also detoxing, pages 112–113). By only juicing, you are depriving your body of essential nutrients vital for recovery, repair, and overall health, such as protein, fiber, calcium, and healthy fats.

● **Soy** Fear of eating soy, especially with hormone-positive breast cancers, stems from the idea that phytoestrogen compounds in soybeans have estrogen-like properties. However, plant-based estrogens are chemically different from human. In fact, research on consumption of soy foods and cancer (though limited), suggests that eating whole soybean products like tofu, tempeh, edamame, soy milk, or similar may actually have a positive impact on overall mortality and prevention of breast cancer.

● **Fasting** Some animal studies have found fasting may have the potential to enhance chemotherapy. There have been a few human studies, but not enough to warrant suggesting fasting as an aid to cancer treatment. Fasting can carry many risks, especially if you're diabetic, have a history of an eating disorder, a low BMI, or you have lost more than 10 percent of weight in the preceding year.

Could supplements help?

IN MOST CASES, SUPPLEMENTS ARE NOT AS EFFECTIVE AS A BALANCED DIET.
Vitamin D supplements can help to support the immune system, especially if access to sunshine is limited. You should continue to take supplements needed for dietary requirements, such as vitamin B12 for vegans, which helps keep blood cells healthy. If appetite is low or you're experiencing diarrhea and/or vomiting, and it's difficult to eat, nutrient supplementation can be arranged often via liquids. Always check with your oncologist because some supplements may interfere with cancer treatments.

Busting the "alkaline diet" myth

The "alkaline diet" is based on a mistaken belief that the acidity or alkalinity of blood can greatly fluctuate and that what we eat can impact on the pH of blood. In reality, the body keeps blood pH within a tight range, and the mechanisms for doing so have nothing to do with digestion.

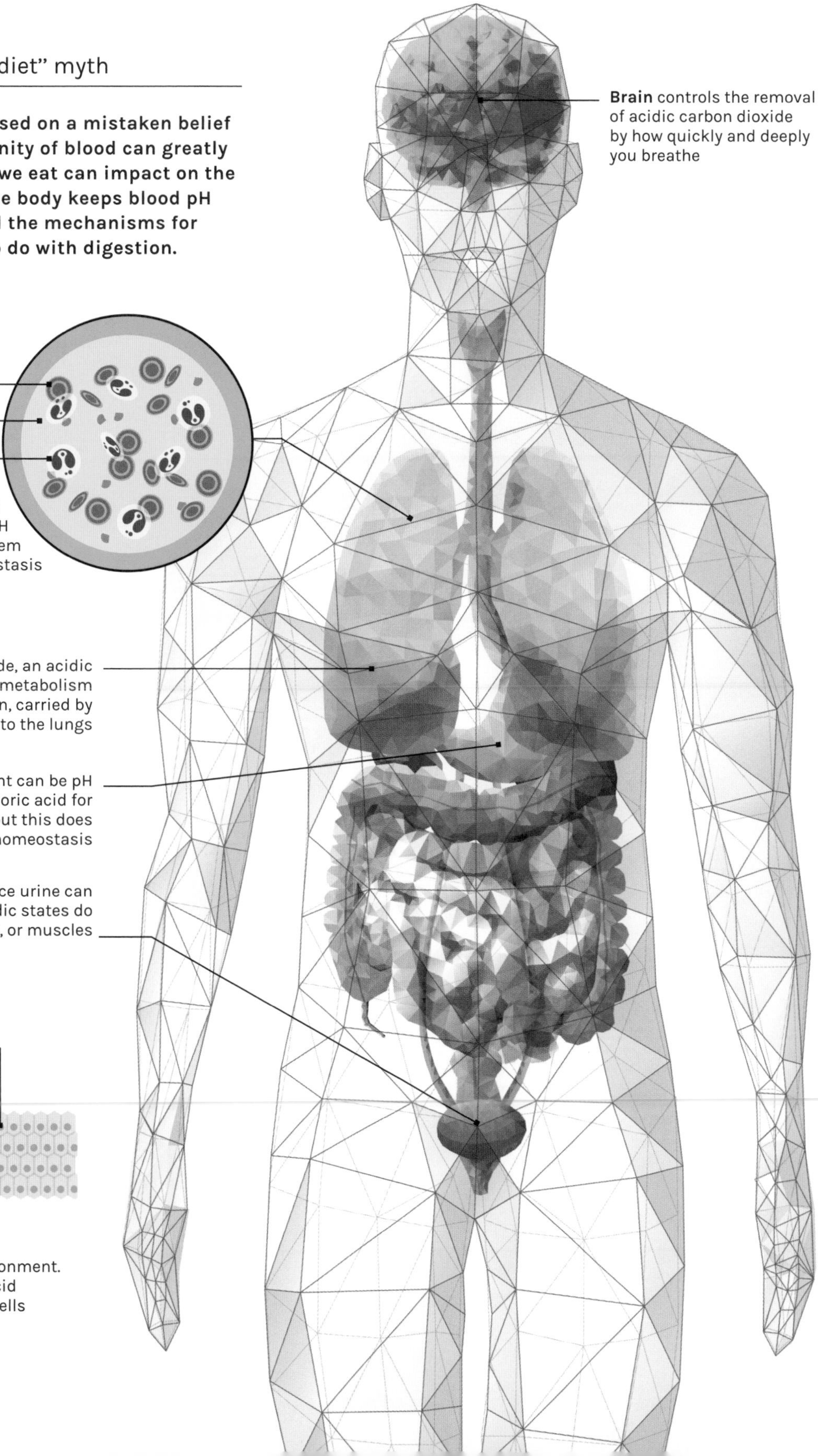

Brain controls the removal of acidic carbon dioxide by how quickly and deeply you breathe

red blood cells

plasma

white blood cells

Blood is maintained at a slightly alkaline pH 7.36– 7.44 through a system of acid-base homeostasis

Lungs expel carbon dioxide, an acidic waste product from the metabolism of nutrients and oxygen, carried by blood from cells to the lungs

Stomach environment can be pH 2–3.5 due to hydrochloric acid for breaking down food, but this does not impact acid-base homeostasis

Kidneys excrete acidity, hence urine can be more acidic, but these acidic states do not get into our brain, blood, or muscles

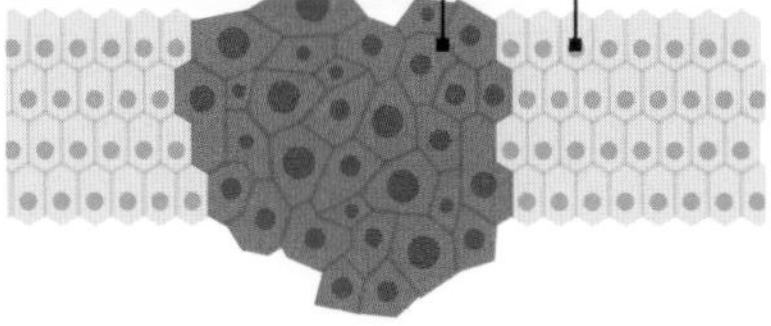

normal cells

cancer cells

Cancer cells create acid environment. Growth rate increases in an acid environment, but the cancer cells themselves create the acid.

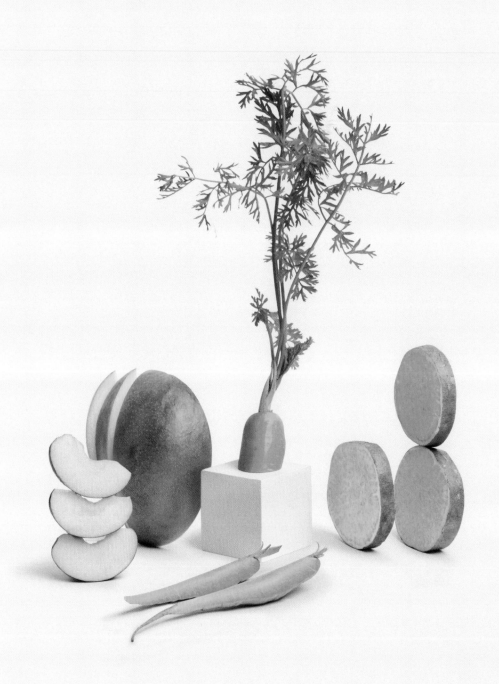

HOW DOES NUTRITION AFFECT CHILD DEVELOPMENT?

CAN DIET IMPROVE FERTILITY?

Diet can improve fertility in both men and women. What you eat affects the quality of sperm and eggs and regulates hormones, including those that facilitate pregnancy. But other lifestyle factors are also crucial.

———————

Getting pregnant isn't as simple as it sounds. Multiple factors can affect fertility, including stress or lack of exercise or sleep. Along with a good diet, people wanting to maximize their fertility need a lot of fresh air, exercise, and rest.

If you smoke, stop! It is linked to reduced fertility in both women and men. Also, avoid or reduce caffeine (stick to 1–2 cups per day at most), and avoid alcohol altogether.

Exercise is important not just because it promotes physical vigor and mental health but also because it helps maintain a healthy body weight, which could improve fertility.

In women, being very low or high in weight can impact fertility. At the higher end of the spectrum, excess fat increases estrogen levels, which could lead to irregular cycles and missed ovulation. At the low end, the body may shut down the reproductive system to preserve fuel for essential body processes.

In men, obesity affects the molecular and physical structure of sperm and is linked to reduced fertility.

HOW TO EAT

A varied and balanced diet promotes fertility. Keep in mind the two Qs—quality and quantity. Focus on nutritional content and the portion that's right for you, rather than the number of calories.

I am an advocate of the Mediterranean diet (see pages 36–39)—minus the red wine for women. Research indicates that women with this pattern of eating have a 66 percent lower risk of experiencing infertility.

Women should supplement their diet with folic acid (see left) and vitamin D during the winter months (or all year round if sun exposure is limited). Take 10µg daily from September to March.

Men can improve sperm quality by including meat, shellfish, nuts, and whole grains in their diet (the Mediterranean diet incorporates these). Bear in mind that a high intake of processed and red meat by men has been shown to reduce rates of conception.

Certain nutrients are known to influence fertility in men. The body requires selenium (found in Brazil nuts, fish, meat, and eggs) to make healthy sperm. Low levels of zinc have been linked to reduced testosterone levels, so it's important to keep zinc levels topped off, preferably through diet. Omega-3 fatty acids, found in oily fish, help produce prostaglandins, compounds that are important for making sperm.

Folate and folic acid

IT'S IMPORTANT FOR WOMEN TO CONSUME DIETARY FOLATE AND ALSO SUPPLEMENT DURING PRECONCEPTION AND EARLY PREGNANCY.
Folate (vitamin B9) improves the quality and maturation of eggs, helps the body make healthy blood cells, and enables an embryo's brain, skull, and spinal cord to develop properly (avoiding neural tube defects such as spina bifida). Ensure your diet is rich in folate, which is found in dark green leafy veggies like broccoli and spinach and in many legumes, including chickpeas. Folic acid is the synthetic version. If planning to conceive, build up stores by taking a 400mcg dose daily three months before you begin trying. Continue supplementing until week 12 of pregnancy.

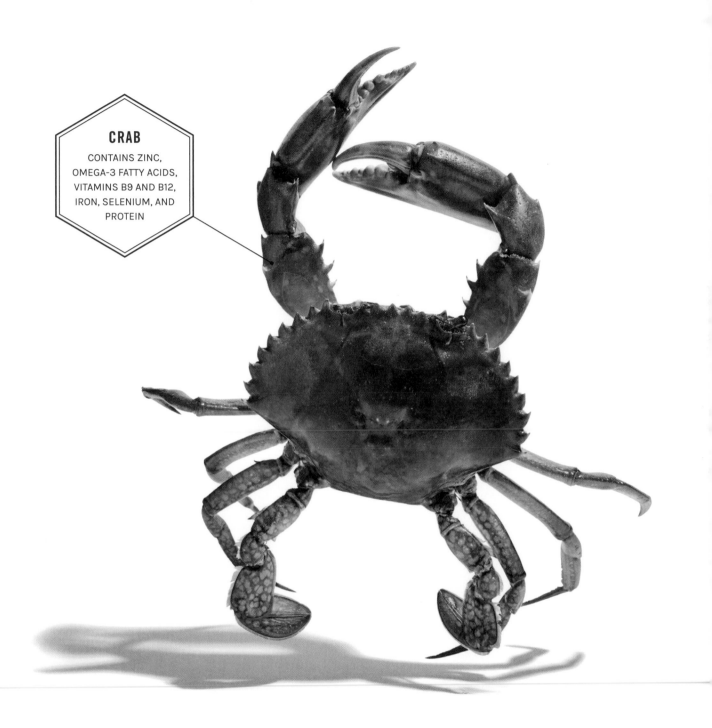

CRAB
CONTAINS ZINC,
OMEGA-3 FATTY ACIDS,
VITAMINS B9 AND B12,
IRON, SELENIUM, AND
PROTEIN

Shellfish like crab contain zinc, which is vital
for DNA repair and function and improves
sperm quality. Low levels are associated with
reduce levels of testosterone in men.

WHY IS NUTRITION SO IMPORTANT DURING PREGNANCY?

Leading child health experts worldwide agree that care given from conception to a child's second birthday—the first 1,000 days—has more influence on a child's future than any other time in their life, and this includes what the mother's diet looks like.

A mother's diet and her nutrient stores are the only source of nutrition for a developing baby, so it is critical that women get the health care and nutritious food they need before and during pregnancy.

CRUCIAL TRIMESTERS

During the three trimesters of pregnancy, a woman's diet, weight fluctuations, physical and mental well-being, environment, and lifestyle habits can have a huge impact on her child's future health. These factors influence how a child's metabolism, immune system, and organ function begin to develop, not to mention the outcome of whether a child is born prematurely or at a low birth weight, which may have a lasting impact on a child's health well into adulthood. The vitamins, nutrients, and calorie intake needed vary depending on the trimester.

A growing body of research suggests that diseases later in life such as diabetes, hypertension, and stroke have their origins in the womb—and that prenatal nutrition plays an important role in whether a child becomes susceptible to these and other illnesses later in life.

But pregnancy can be tough: aversions to food, no appetite, a large appetite, reflux, sickness—you name it; most women will have some kind of food challenge throughout those nine months when the baby is growing. The good news is that as long as you avoid certain risky foods and drinks (see pages 182–185), enjoy a generally healthy diet and lifestyle, and pay attention to particular nutrients that are key to a baby's development—especially their brain (see below and right)—you should have little to worry about.

Building the brain

The following key nutrients have been studied and linked with development of the baby's brain in the womb. Before taking supplements, speak to a health professional.

CHOLINE

FOOD SOURCES

EGGS | LEAN MEATS | POULTRY | CRUCIFEROUS VEGETABLES (BRASSICAS) | NUTS | LEGUMES

SHOULD I SUPPLEMENT?

Supplementing with twice the recommended amount of choline (930mg/day) in the third trimester of pregnancy may improve speed of processing in infants; especially important for plant-based eaters.

VITAMIN D

FOOD SOURCES

Limited but include oily fish, egg yolks, meat and offal, fortified foods, and mushrooms grown in sunlight (see pages 138-139).

SHOULD I SUPPLEMENT?

If you get little or no sun exposure, take a daily 10mcg supplement all year. Deficiency in pregnancy has been linked to an increased risk of a child developing ADHD and a reduction in IQ and language abilities.

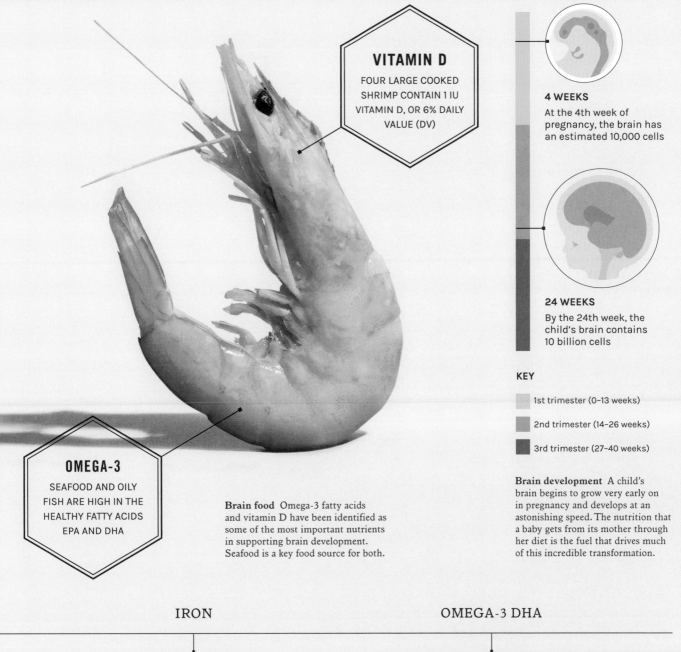

VITAMIN D

FOUR LARGE COOKED SHRIMP CONTAIN 1 IU VITAMIN D, OR 6% DAILY VALUE (DV)

4 WEEKS

At the 4th week of pregnancy, the brain has an estimated 10,000 cells

24 WEEKS

By the 24th week, the child's brain contains 10 billion cells

KEY

1st trimester (0–13 weeks)

2nd trimester (14–26 weeks)

3rd trimester (27–40 weeks)

OMEGA-3

SEAFOOD AND OILY FISH ARE HIGH IN THE HEALTHY FATTY ACIDS EPA AND DHA

Brain food Omega-3 fatty acids and vitamin D have been identified as some of the most important nutrients in supporting brain development. Seafood is a key food source for both.

Brain development A child's brain begins to grow very early on in pregnancy and develops at an astonishing speed. The nutrition that a baby gets from its mother through her diet is the fuel that drives much of this incredible transformation.

IRON

FOOD SOURCES

SHELLFISH | BROCCOLI | RED MEAT | TOFU
NUTS | BEANS | DRIED FRUIT

SHOULD I SUPPLEMENT?

Up to 50 percent of pregnant women are iron deficient, which may cause irreversible neural issues in the fetus; those with gestational diabetes are more at risk. Iron in the third trimester is especially important.

OMEGA-3 DHA

FOOD SOURCES

FISH AND SEAFOOD | SEAWEED AND ALGAE

SHOULD I SUPPLEMENT?

A fetus's needs increase sharply in the third trimester since the brain consists of fatty acids. Some studies suggest DHA supplements could give babies better memory, attention, and verbal skills, and a lower risk of neurological disorders.

WHAT FOODS SHOULD I AVOID DURING PREGNANCY?

Pregnancy can be a very exciting but also anxious time for expectant moms, with many conflicting messages on the internet or from others on what you should and shouldn't be eating. So what is safe, and what is not?

Most foods that pregnant women are advised to avoid carry a risk of food poisoning from harmful bacteria when undercooked or prepared in a certain way. The current US guidelines are as follows:

PREPARED FOOD

● **Premade deli salads:** Don't buy or eat premade ham salad, chicken salad, or seafood salad, which may contain *Listeria*—bacteria that can cause an infection called listeriosis, which can harm a fetus or newborn. These items are commonly found in delis.

● **Unwashed packaged salad:** It is fine to eat preprepared, prewashed salad if you keep it in the fridge and eat it before the use-by date. Avoid eating raw sprouts of any kind (including alfalfa, clover, radish, and mung bean).

● **Pâté:** Avoid all types of pâté, as they may contain *Listeria*.

DAIRY AND EGGS

● **Unpasteurized milk and dairy:** Most milk and dairy products, including cheese, sold in the US are pasteurized and safe to consume—but avoid unpasteurized (raw) milk and dairy. If you only have access to unpasteurized milk, boil it before using.

● **Raw or undercooked eggs:** Cook eggs until the yolks and whites are firm. If you are making a casserole or other dish containing eggs, make sure the dish is cooked to a temperature of 160°F. Try to avoid foods that contain raw egg, such as homemade mayonnaise or mousse. Make sure that foods that contain raw or lightly cooked eggs are made only with pasteurized eggs.

MEAT

● **Raw or undercooked meat:** Avoid any undercooked meat, especially poultry, pork, sausages, and burgers. Meat should always be

---

Which cheeses can I eat?

SAFE TO EAT

Some cheeses are safe to eat when pregnant, but not all of them, as some contain unpasteurized dairy and are more susceptible to bacterial growth. This breakdown shows which types are safe and which are best to avoid.

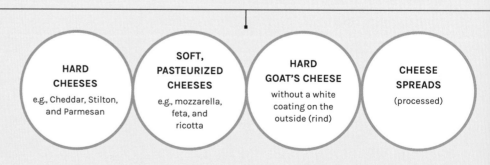

HARD CHEESES
e.g., Cheddar, Stilton, and Parmesan

SOFT, PASTEURIZED CHEESES
e.g., mozzarella, feta, and ricotta

HARD GOAT'S CHEESE
without a white coating on the outside (rind)

CHEESE SPREADS
(processed)

cooked thoroughly and not be pink or bloody, as there is a risk of toxoplasmosis, a parasitic infection that can be harmful to you and your baby.

It's safe to eat cold, prepackaged meat such as ham. You may prefer to avoid raw cured meats; if not, freeze for four days before defrosting or eat them cooked. Avoid game, as it may contain lead shot.

FISH

- **Some fish:** Pregnant women should eat a diverse diet that includes 8-12oz of low-mercury fish weekly to help boost omega-3 consumption. All seafood dishes should be cooked to 145°F.

- **Raw shellfish:** Cooked shellfish is safe, but raw shellfish can cause food poisoning.

Vitamin A

TOO MUCH VITAMIN A CAN BE HARMFUL TO AN UNBORN BABY, POTENTIALLY LEADING TO BIRTH DEFECTS AND EVEN MISCARRIAGE. Avoid liver and liver products and multivitamins containing vitamin A or fish liver oils. It's fine to eat foods that naturally contain low levels of vitamin A, like carrots, but avoid any that have vitamin A added. Cosmetic products, like face cream, that contain vitamin A are safe to use.

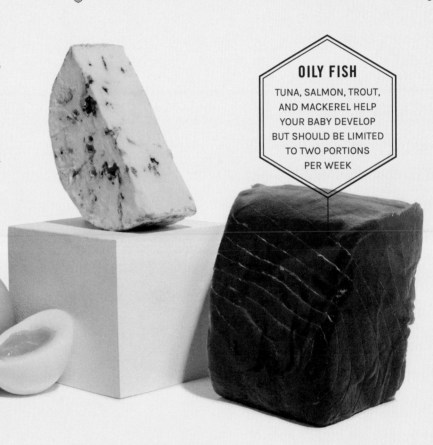

OILY FISH

TUNA, SALMON, TROUT, AND MACKEREL HELP YOUR BABY DEVELOP BUT SHOULD BE LIMITED TO TWO PORTIONS PER WEEK

RAW EGGS

RAW EGGS ARE BEST AVOIDED AS THEY COULD CONTAIN SALMONELLA BACTERIA, WHICH CAN CAUSE FOOD POISONING

AVOID UNLESS COOKED

Avoid these types of cheese unless cooked until steaming hot, as they can cause listeriosis.

SOFT, UNPASTEURIZED CHEESES

SOFT BLUE CHEESES e.g., Danish blue, Gorgonzola, and Roquefort

SOFT GOAT'S CHEESE

MOLD -RIPENED SOFT CHEESES with a white coating, e.g., Brie, Camembert, and chèvre

These contain more moisture, making it easier for bacteria to grow

WHY DO WOMEN GET STRANGE FOOD CRAVINGS IN PREGNANCY?

We've all heard stories of the unusual items or food combinations women want to eat while pregnant. In truth, there is very little research on the subject and a lot of old wives' tales.

Some women crave unhealthy items during pregnancy, while the lucky few experience healthier cravings for fruits and vegetables. Others have no appetite at all. We don't know much about why this happens, but cravings may be caused by hormonal changes, physiological changes, or even the emotional roller coaster of pregnancy.

POTENTIAL CAUSES

The nausea and sickness some women experience during pregnancy is incredibly taxing on the body. Sometimes food cravings can materialize as a coping strategy and a way to manage hormonal fluctuations or difficult moments. There has also been talk of women "needing" certain vitamins

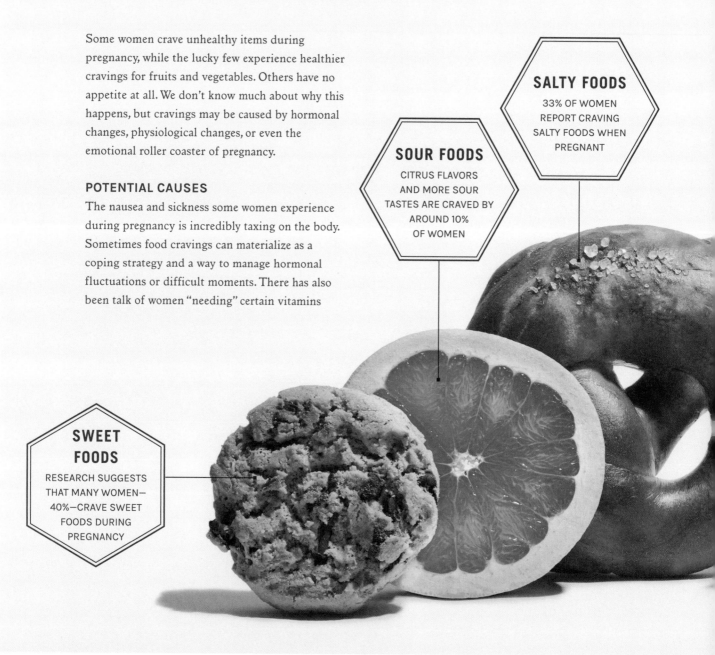

SOUR FOODS
CITRUS FLAVORS AND MORE SOUR TASTES ARE CRAVED BY AROUND 10% OF WOMEN

SALTY FOODS
33% OF WOMEN REPORT CRAVING SALTY FOODS WHEN PREGNANT

SWEET FOODS
RESEARCH SUGGESTS THAT MANY WOMEN—40%—CRAVE SWEET FOODS DURING PREGNANCY

and minerals and therefore craving foods that contain them. However, if you have a craving for less healthy options, it's unlikely that your body is trying to meet a nutritional need. If that were the case, you would be more likely to crave foods such as fish, broccoli, and whole grains, which many in the US don't eat enough of.

BEST PRACTICE

It's good to be aware of what your body is telling you, but it's also important not to always give in to food cravings, as your diet during pregnancy needs to be varied to provide all the nutrients your baby needs.

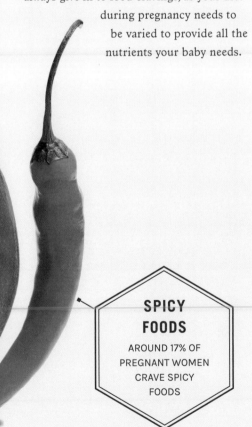

SPICY FOODS

AROUND 17% OF PREGNANT WOMEN CRAVE SPICY FOODS

WHAT SHOULD I DRINK DURING PREGNANCY?

Staying hydrated is vital during pregnancy. You'll need seven to 10 glasses of fluid a day—possibly more if you're active or the weather is hot—but be mindful of what you are drinking.

———

Try to get your fluid intake from a variety of sources. Remember your limits with each type (see below) and avoid too many sugary drinks, as flavor preferences can be developed in the womb (see pages 186–187).

LIMIT CAFFEINE

The National Institutes of Health (NIH) warns that too much caffeine can result in miscarriage or a low birth weight. The NIH advises pregnant women to drink no more than two mugs of regular coffee, or less than 200mg of caffeine, per day. Research suggests that the amount of caffeine in coffee can range from 50mg per cup to more than 300mg, while other foods, such as chocolate, and medications also contain caffeine, so it would be easy to exceed the recommended limit without realizing. Ask about caffeine content before you buy. If unknown, it is best to avoid. Note also that green tea contains up to 100mg caffeine, and some herbal teas may not be fully safe in large amounts.

AVOID ALCOHOL

It is safest to avoid alcohol completely during pregnancy; it has been linked to low birth weight, premature birth, and miscarriage. It can also affect a baby's development and long-term health. Experts cannot be sure that any amount of alcohol is safe, but drinking heavily during pregnancy can result in your baby developing fetal alcohol syndrome (FAS), a serious condition with symptoms including growth, learning, and behavioral issues. If you are finding it difficult to stop drinking, ask for support from your midwife or OB.

DO A CHILD'S FOOD PREFERENCES DEVELOP IN THE WOMB?

There has been a lot of research into the nutrition a baby receives from its mother inside the womb and through breast milk, and the results are fascinating.

———————

Research suggests that babies start to develop preferences for certain flavors in the womb, delivered via the amniotic fluid, and then via breastfeeding, with potential implications for lifelong eating habits. It is a tricky area to research ethically when it comes to a poor diet and the impact on a baby's future health, but we know that the most researched flavors that are easily available in amniotic fluid and breast milk are garlic, carrot, alcohol, anise, and vanilla.

PUNGENT GARLIC
FLAVOR COMES FROM THE COMPOUND ALLICIN, WHICH ONLY FORMS WHEN CLOVES ARE CRUSHED.

INNATE PREFERENCES

Around 16 weeks after conception, fetuses develop pores on their taste buds that allow them to identify basic tastes, and they will swallow more amniotic fluid when it's sweet and less when it's bitter. Penchants for salt and umami tastes are also innate. Available data suggests that infants are born "hard-wired" to prefer tastes that signal beneficial nutrients (for example, sweet tastes signal calories) and to reject tastes that signal harmful compounds (for example, bitter tastes signal poison).

LEARNED PREFERENCES

Most of our food preferences, however, are learned, and a growing body of research shows that this learning also begins before birth. From as early as 21 weeks old the fetus can detect complex flavors,

Early exposure Babies can detect particularly strong flavors such as garlic in amniotic fluid and breast milk and can develop preferences accordingly.

such as garlic and carrot, a few hours after the mother has eaten those foods. This can result in preferences for these flavors at birth through breast milk and weaning. For example, babies who tasted high concentrations of carrot in utero and in their mother's milk went on to happily eat more carrots during weaning. However, this has also been shown to ring true with unhealthy items. The more little ones are exposed in the womb to less healthy foods, the more desensitized they may become to it when older, meaning they may eat more cake, chocolate, and chips to get the same reward centers to light up.

BEST PRACTICE

It makes sense to eat a varied diet when pregnant and nursing to enhance the likelihood that your baby will eat a wider variety of foods, but fear not if this has not been an option for you. There is ample opportunity to improve this during the weaning stage (see pages 194–195). Exposing your baby to a variety of novel foods in infancy will reduce the likelihood of them developing a neophobia or aversion to foods later on in life.

Taste development in unborn babies

Taste and flavor perception are central to the development of food preferences. Both begin in the womb due to changes in the gustatory and olfactory system, beginning in the first trimester of pregnancy.

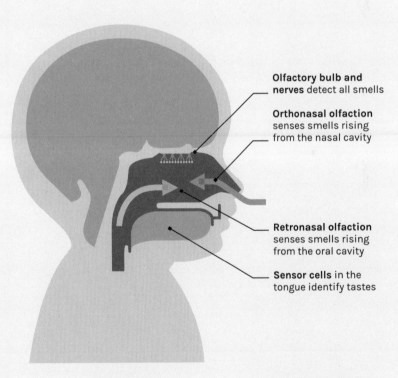

Olfactory bulb and nerves detect all smells

Orthonasal olfaction senses smells rising from the nasal cavity

Retronasal olfaction senses smells rising from the oral cavity

Sensor cells in the tongue identify tastes

THE FIVE BASIC TASTES

Taste sensations result from activation of the gustatory system—taste cells in the mouth, neural pathways, and the gustatory cortex in the brain—and are limited to sweet, bitter, sour, salty, and umami.

A MYRIAD OF ODORS

Thousands of different odors stimulate the olfactory bulb and nerves in the nasal cavity to create smell sensations.

THE SYNTHESIS OF FLAVOR

Flavor perception then results from the integration of the taste and smell sensory systems. Odors sensed orthonasally and retronasally combine with tastes detected in the oral cavity to create flavor sensations.

WILL MY CHILD DEVELOP FOOD ALLERGIES?

Food allergies affect 32 million Americans, including 5.6 million children under age 18. That's about 1 in 13 children, or two in every classroom.

Importantly, if you have a food allergy, that doesn't mean your baby will, but there is a higher chance of that allergy being present, as the likelihood can be down to genetics. If a parent or sibling has a food allergy or eczema or asthma, the risk increases for a child to have a food allergy.

DURING PREGNANCY

There is no firm evidence that eliminating certain foods from the diet during pregnancy has any impact on the development of future allergies; it may even have a detrimental effect, causing deficiencies in key nutrients for mother or baby. Some research has suggested that taking omega-3 supplements may reduce the risk, but the results are not conclusive.

DURING INFANCY

While there is no one food or diet that can eliminate the risk of an allergy, it is thought that exclusively breastfeeding for the first six months of the baby's life can reduce the risk. Some allergies, such as eggs and milk, can disappear as a child grows up, but some, like peanuts, can be lifelong. If you have any concerns, speak to your health professional before starting to wean.

PEANUT ALLERGIES

In the US, peanuts are deemed safe to eat during pregnancy. Government advice used to be to avoid giving foods containing peanuts to children under three, but the latest research shows no clear evidence that this reduces the risk and may in fact increase risk (see below), so peanuts—ground or in a butter due to the risk of choking on whole nuts—should not be avoided, unless the child has a known allergy.

Should I take probiotics?

SOME RESEARCH SUGGESTS THAT TAKING A PROBIOTIC SUPPLEMENT IN PREGNANCY CAN REDUCE THE RISK OF THE BABY DEVELOPING A FOOD ALLERGY. However, more research is needed and there are no current guidelines for pregnant women on which probiotic to choose, so be cautious when taking any supplements.

LEAP peanut study

A LEAP study looked at peanut allergies in children, as numbers have risen in the last 10 years. They recruited 640 babies aged 4–11 months with eczema and/or an egg allergy, as this increases the risk of having a peanut allergy. Results showed a reduced risk in babies who ate peanuts.

ATE PEANUTS	AVOIDED PEANUTS
The babies who were assigned to consume peanuts had a	The babies who avoided peanuts had a
3.2%	**17.2%**
chance of developing a peanut allergy	chance of developing a peanut allergy

SHOULD I CHANGE MY NUTRITION AFTER GIVING BIRTH?

The period after giving birth is an opportunity for the mother to be looked after and to recover. Key to that process is making sure she gets the right nutrition.

Keeping up with the demands of feeding while sleep-deprived and trying to recover from the birth is hard. For many women, it can take several months to adjust. To help restore health, replenish nutrient stores, and, if breastfeeding, support lactation, new mothers should eat nourishing foods that meet their body's changing needs.

POSTPARTUM NUTRITION

New moms should eat and drink regularly, following a healthy, balanced diet. This should include lots of fruits and vegetables, as well as proteins to help the body recover, fiber-rich carbohydrates for energy, and iron-rich foods to help create new blood cells—especially if the mother has anemia or lost a lot of blood during the birth. They will need on average between 1,800 and 2,200 calories a day, and 500 calories more than this if breastfeeding.

NUTRIENTS FOR BREASTFEEDING

Breastfeeding moms should limit their intake of alcohol and caffeine, as these can pass into breast milk and affect the baby's digestion, sleep, and feeding. They should also be aware of the following additional nutritional needs during this period:

● **Increased calcium:** An extra 550mg per day is required to support milk production and replenish calcium stores. Include calcium-rich foods in your diet, e.g., milk, cheese, yogurts. If your diet is plant-based (see pages 116–133), choose calcium-enriched options.

● **Increased zinc:** An extra 4mg per day is required if breastfeeding. Zinc supports the immune system and is found in beef, fish, beans, tofu, nuts, and seeds.

● **Omega-3s:** Evidence suggests that a diet rich in omega-3s results in omega-3-rich breast milk, which supports brain development in babies. Sources include some nuts and seeds and oily fish (see pages 184–185).

● **Increased fluids:** You will need to drink more fluids, remembering to do so before a headache begins. The amount needed will vary, but the Institute of Medicine recommends 14–16 cups of water per day.

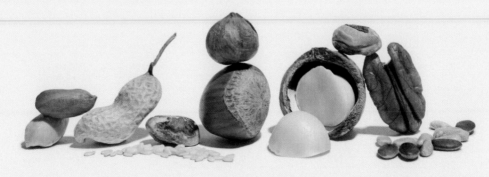

HOW CAN I GIVE MY CHILD THE BEST NUTRITIONAL START?

Once born, babies reach a range of milestones as they continue to grow and develop, but it's important to provide them with the right nutrition to do so from day one.

Exclusive breastfeeding for the first six months of a baby's life is recommended, as the mother's milk contains all the nutrients her infant needs. But if this isn't possible, formula—which mimics the nutrition of breast milk—should be used instead. It's important to note that however you decide to feed your baby is *your* choice.

BREASTFEEDING

Breastfeeding is the most nutritious, cost-effective, and often the most convenient option for feeding a baby. Breast milk contains a variety of nutrients and proteins, as well as growth factors, antibodies, and hormones vital to a baby's development that cannot be replicated in infant formula. Breast milk and the process of feeding is also critical to the seeding of a baby's gut microbiome (see pages 140–141). Thanks to the mother-to-child interaction, breastfeeding also plays an important role in strengthening a baby's sensory and emotional circuitry, critical for cognitive and socio-emotional development. Research also suggests breastfeeding may lower the mother's risk of developing breast cancer, ovarian cancer, cardiovascular disease, osteoporosis, and obesity.

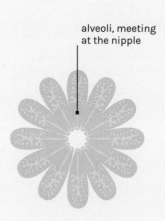

alveoli, meeting at the nipple

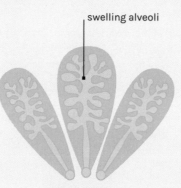

swelling alveoli

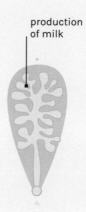

production of milk

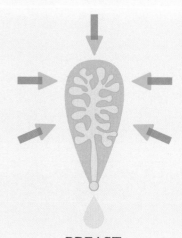

How breast milk is made

Hormonal changes caused by the different stages of pregnancy and birth kick-start the production of breast milk.

DURING PREGNANCY

Estrogen and progesterone levels increase during pregnancy, stimulating the alveoli cells and milk ducts in the breast to grow

AT BIRTH

Prolactin hormone, released once the baby is born, triggers the alveoli cells to produce milk

BREAST FEEDING

Oxytocin hormone is released when the baby suckles, causing the muscles around the alveoli cells to squeeze the milk out of the milk ducts in the nipple— known as the let-down reflex

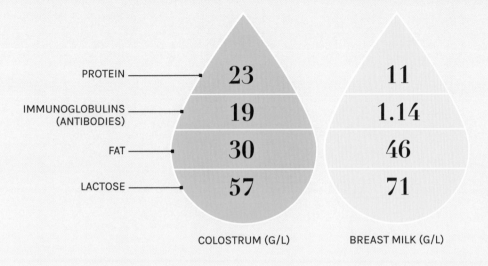

PROTEIN — **23**

IMMUNOGLOBULINS — **19**
(ANTIBODIES)

FAT — **30**

LACTOSE — **57**

COLOSTRUM (G/L)

11

1.14

46

71

BREAST MILK (G/L)

Colostrum and breast milk compared Thick, yellow colostrum is high in protein and antibodies. Mature breast milk is high in water, fat, and lactose.

WHAT IS COLOSTRUM?

The first milk a mother produces in the days after giving birth is literally golden—it's called colostrum and is particularly rich and concentrated to give the baby the best possible start.

Colostrum is packed with protein, antibodies, and vitamins A, D, and B12, which are all important in supporting the baby's growth and immune system.

After a few days, the mother begins to produce "mature" breast milk, which is less concentrated and lower in protein and antibodies than colostrum but higher in fat and lactose (see above).

THE BENEFITS OF BREAST MILK

As well as providing essential nutrition from protein, lactose, fats, vitamins, and minerals, breast milk boasts numerous other health benefits.

Breastfeeding transfers vital antibodies from mother to child to support their immune system, reducing the risk of illness and sudden infant death syndrome (SIDS), as well as that of obesity and cardiovascular disease in adulthood.

Many of the body's hormones, which are vital for regulating bodily functions, growth, appetite, and weight, are transmitted from mother to baby through breast milk. Studies have shown that breast milk contains diverse gut bacteria, which transfer to the baby via breastfeeding and areolar skin contact, seeding a healthy gut microbiome.

FORMULA

For a variety of reasons, breastfeeding may not be an option for you, and there is absolutely no need to feel guilty about that—it does not mean your baby has to miss out. Formula milks today have been designed to give all the key nutrition babies need. Formula comes fortified with essential vitamins, so whereas all breastfed babies should be given a daily supplement of vitamin D (400 IU) from birth, babies who are given more than 17oz (500ml) of infant formula a day do not need this.

CHANGES AT SIX MONTHS

At six months, a baby's stores of nutrients such as iron, start to deplete, so guidelines recommend that weaning (the introduction of "solid" foods; see pages 192–193) should start at around this time. The American Academy of Pediatrics recommends that exclusively or mostly breastfed babies be given an iron supplement starting at 4 months of age. Talk to your baby's healthcare provider about supplementation.

WHAT ARE THE BEST STRATEGIES FOR WEANING?

A baby's first taste experiences can set them up for a great relationship with food. Traditionally, babies are given fruit purées as first foods, but research suggests that offering a variety of flavors encourages an acceptance of variety.

———————

There's nothing wrong with the fruit-purées-first approach. Babies have an innate preference for sweet foods (see page 194). I suggest making weaning all about experimentation and exposure to lots of foods to help your child become accustomed to as many flavors as possible. If you start weaning with savory flavors, you enable your child to learn to accept them and enjoy savory foods before they have a chance to associate solid food very firmly with sweet flavors (which they are predisposed to, as the flavor of milk is sweet). This vegetable-led approach to weaning is by no means the only way to wean, but it is backed by scientific research that shows it can have a positive influence on vegetable intake.

Research suggests that, between the ages of 6 and 12 months, babies are most likely to accept new foods. This gives you the ideal window to introduce a variety of foods into your baby's diet. This nutritional input will support their development, and the familiarity with multiple flavors will help set them up with good dietary habits for life.

Regardless of the method you choose, repeated exposure is vital, so be patient. It can take more than 10 attempts with the same food for it to become accepted regularly. Just keep offering.

And remember, babies have off days, too. Your baby won't want the same amount of food every day. Heat, teething, sickness, and tiredness all affect appetite.

PURÉES OR FINGER FOODS?

Parents following a baby-led approach to weaning bypass purées and offer finger foods from the start, encouraging their baby to feed themselves (once they can sit upright and have the coordination).

Although introducing both purées and finger foods into the diet together has received mixed feedback, it may actually help babies develop

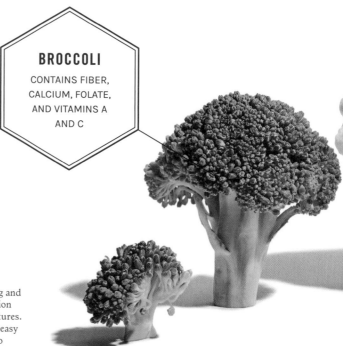

BROCCOLI
CONTAINS FIBER, CALCIUM, FOLATE, AND VITAMINS A AND C

Finger foods encourage self-feeding and help babies improve their coordination and become accustomed to new textures. Broccoli and cauliflower "trees" are easy to pick up and have great textures to stimulate your baby's mouth.

coordination and independence and discover what they like to eat best. Some people wrongly believe that offering a spoon alongside finger foods may confuse a baby and cause them to choke.

Finger foods have to be soft enough for babies to squash them with their gums and reduce the risk of choking. Ensure rough skin and hard pieces are removed. So if offering zucchini fingers, remove the skin unless it is super soft. With cucumber, offer just the seeds at the center.

When making purées, steam and then blend the food. The texture of early purées should be watery, like milk, then work up gradually to thicker, lumpier consistencies. Think of this as a gradual transition from puréed to mashed to minced to chopped.

MEALTIME ROUTINES

Babies thrive on routine. Within reason, try to feed your baby at the same times each day. You could play music to help build a positive association with meals. A pleasant routine can be reassuring, allowing you to expose your baby to new foods in a comfortable way.

Bitter flavors

INTRODUCING FOODS WITH BITTER FLAVORS EARLY ON MAY BE A GOOD IDEA FOR YOUR CHILD'S LONG-TERM HEALTH.
Research suggests that the phytonutrients found in bitter vegetables may help prevent heart disease and cancer. Try introducing more bitter veggies, like broccoli or Brussels sprouts, alongside less intensely flavored veggies like cauliflower, to encourage your baby to develop an acceptance of and a liking for their flavors and textures.

Eat together when you can. Good role modeling can encourage your baby to eat more and try new foods. They will even learn by watching you chew and swallow food.

Stay positive and calm. Don't let your baby's facial expressions affect you. Imagine experiencing a food for the first time—it's likely to produce a reaction. This is the wonder of weaning!

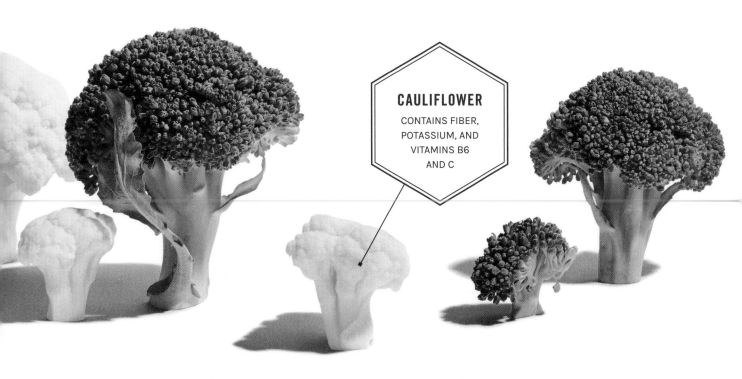

CAULIFLOWER

CONTAINS FIBER, POTASSIUM, AND VITAMINS B6 AND C

HOW DO I PREVENT MY CHILD FROM BECOMING A PICKY EATER?

A young child's relationship with food matters. Picky eaters get less protein, vegetables, and fruits, and research shows that children who don't eat well at the age of three are more likely to remain picky into adulthood.

The phrase "picky eating" describes many behaviors, including the rejection of one or more foods, the limited intake or variety of foods, and/or frequent changes in food preferences. Causes can be difficult to pinpoint. Studies suggest some children are predisposed to food pickiness, just as others are more shy. Many studies show that children respond to their parents' relationships with food, which gives parents the power to influence their child's diet.

THINGS YOU CAN DO

Follow the advice for weaning on pages 192–193 to establish good eating habits early. As often as possible, eat together. Give your child the same food as the rest of the family (minus the salt). The best way for them to learn to eat and enjoy new foods is to copy you. Give your child small portions and a lot of praise for eating, even if it's only a little. If they reject a food, don't force them to eat it. Just take it away without saying anything and try it again another time. Changing how you serve a food may make it more appealing. For instance, a child might refuse cooked carrots but enjoy raw grated carrot.

Your child may be a slow eater, so be patient. Make mealtimes enjoyable and not just about eating. Sit down and chat about other things to give them a chance to finish eating at their own pace.

Don't give your child too many snacks— two healthy snacks a day is plenty. And don't leave meals until your child is too hungry or tired to eat.

If you know kids who are good eaters, ask them over for a meal to set an example—but don't openly compare them to your child. If there is an adult your child looks up to in your life, have them over to eat often. Sometimes a child will eat without fuss around a grandparent, for example.

WHAT NOT TO DO

Avoid showing your child a reaction if they exhibit picky behavior. Try to stay calm, even if it's very frustrating. Reserve all your attention for verbally praising your child whenever they eat well.

Also avoid offering your child overwhelmingly huge portions. Stick with small portions, adding seconds if required.

Natural sweet tooth

THE PREFERENCE BABIES AND YOUNG CHILDREN SHOW FOR SWEET FLAVORS MAY BE DUE TO THE PAIN AND STRESS RELIEF THEY PROVIDE.
In studies, 3-4-month-old babies instantly felt calmer and more trusting around a new face when consuming something sweet. We are hardwired to enjoy sweet foods. They trigger the "feel-good" reward center in the brain and offer a plentiful supply of energy. As we age, our feel-good receptors don't work as efficiently—we grow out of our sweet tooth. That being said, it's important to set up good eating habits early. Offer kids sweet foods in moderation, ideally after establishing savory foods in the diet (see page 192). Avoid offering added sugars (see page 64) to children under two.

Don't leave your child to eat alone. If you can't eat together, stay with them while they eat their own meal.

Avoid using food as a reward. Your child may start to think of sweets as good and vegetables as bad, which can spiral into an unhealthy relationship with food. Instead, reward them with a trip to the park or promise to play a game with them.

It's tempting to give kids things you know they will eat, and ultra-processed foods are highly palatable. Kids might reject foods consistently or eat them only sometimes. Be patient with this and play the long game. While a bag of chips can guarantee the same flavor at each bite and a child that will happily eat what you give them, in the long run, it may create a preference for less healthy foods that becomes a tricky habit to break.

VITAMIN A

CARROTS ARE A GREAT SOURCE OF VITAMIN A, NEEDED TO SUPPORT EYE HEALTH AND THE IMMUNE SYSTEM

Sweet, mild-flavored carrots are a popular choice for transitioning babies to solid food from six months old, but don't be afraid to try more strongly flavored vegetables to help expand your baby's palate.

HOW CAN I HELP MY TODDLER EAT WELL?

Toddlers are notorious for being up and down with their food, and this is completely normal. You need to support and guide your toddler to make the right nutritional choices, which can impact growth, development, and future health outcomes.

From ages one to three, a toddler will be learning to eat with hands and cutlery, in a variety of settings, and manage energy intake for the amount of growing and exploring they will do. Some children will eat more than others. Teething, sickness, activity levels, and sleep can all impact appetite.

ESTABLISH GOOD HABITS

A positive eating environment at home is key to encouraging good eating behaviors. Get your children involved with cooking so they can see the process from start to finish; sing songs and get creative to make it all the more fun.

Provide your child with exposure to lots of different foods. Don't give up after introducing a new food once—it can take between 5 and 15 times before they will accept a new food. Try to stay as relaxed as possible before and during mealtimes, and be a role model for eating a variety of different foods and having a healthy relationship toward food intake. The more you pressurize your child, the less likely they are to want to try new foods or eat their meal. Limit bribery, as this will only make things more difficult in the long run. For example, avoid saying, "If you eat your greens, you can have dessert," or making a child feel guilty for not eating a food because others elsewhere have less.

Ensure your kitchen and home are full of healthy foods. Utilize the freezer and try batch-cooking a favorite meal with lots of added vegetables. For example, make a cauliflower mac 'n' cheese and include the cauliflower stalk and leaves, along with broccoli, peas, and carrots, and freeze into individual portions for the next few weeks.

A quick guide to nutritional needs,

Each day toddlers need three meals and some snacks made up of the four main food groups, in the right balance and in portion sizes just right for them. For most toddlers, there is no need to offer low-calorie or low-fat options as children of this age need lots of energy for growing and physical activity.

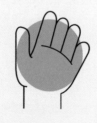

5+
Portions of
FRUITS AND VEGETABLES

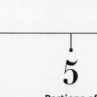

5
Portions of
STARCHY CARBOHYDRATES

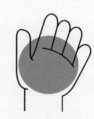

3
Portions of
DAIRY AND ALTERNATIVES

MILK

Quantity?
At least 12oz (350ml) of milk a day OR 2 servings of dairy foods such as cheese or yogurt.

How long?
WHO recommends breastfeeding until 2 years old; offer cow's milk or an alternative after 12 months.

Vegans:
Make sure dairy alternatives are fortified. Avoid rice milk, which contains a level of arsenic too high for toddlers.

SALT

Quantity?
Children aged 1 to 3 years should have no more than 2g of salt (800mg sodium) per day.

Yes or no?
There is no reason to add salt to your child's diet at any age unless you have been advised to do so by your health professional.

SUGAR

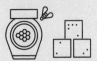

Quantity?
Avoid added sugar, except occasionally from 2+.

Desserts
Include to maximize nutrition, but make it fruit and yogurt or something less sweet.

Drinks
Water and milk are best as they do not contain added sugar. No milk after brushing teeth from 2+.

Snacks
Avoid too much dried fruit as it can get stuck on teeth and cause decay.

FATS & PROTEIN

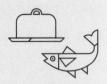

Quantity?
Until the age of 2, children need a lot of energy from fat. After that, lower-fat options can be offered.

Saturated fats
Limit saturated fat to less than 10% of overall daily calories. Steam, grill, or bake foods instead of frying them to reduce saturated fat.

Protein
Replace processed and high-fat meats with beans, peas, and lentils to meet protein needs, but be aware that high-fiber foods may fill little tummies too quickly.

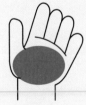

2+
Portions of
PROTEIN
(3 IF VEGETARIAN)

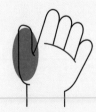

<1
A small amount of
FAT

Should I give my toddler supplements?

GOVERNMENT ADVICE IS THAT CHILDREN AGED SIX MONTHS TO FIVE YEARS OLD SHOULD TAKE A DAILY VITAMIN D SUPPLEMENT
if consuming less than 17oz (500ml) formula milk. However, recently it has been reported that more children are getting enough vitamins in their diets. With the exception of vitamin D, if your child has a balanced diet with lots of color and variety, then they will be getting enough. If you are concerned, ask your doctor for a referral to a pediatric dietitian.

WHAT SHOULD I CONSIDER IF RAISING A CHILD ON A VEGAN OR VEGETARIAN DIET?

Times have changed substantially in the last 20 years, and plant-based diets are on the rise, but what does that mean for little eaters? Is it possible to give them all the nutrition they require from a plant-based diet?

The short answer is "yes," but it needs to be carefully thought through, with potential supplementation provided if on a vegan diet.

NUTRIENT DENSITY FOR VEGANS

For healthy development, a vegan child needs enough calories, healthy fats, and protein. Vegan diets can be high in fiber, which can make toddlers' tummies full without sufficient calories. Guard against this by including energy- and nutrient-dense foods such as avocados, vegetable oils, seeds, nut butters or ground-up nuts (no whole nuts to the age of five, due to choking risk), tofu, and legumes.

PROTEIN CONSIDERATIONS

Protein needs are easily met if your child eats a wide variety of foods containing protein at each meal. From nondairy yogurts to beans, peas, and lentils, to grains like quinoa and buckwheat, to tofu and other soy products, there are many options for vegan and plant-based eaters. Alongside the essential amino acids we should all be consuming (see pages 14–15 and 128–129), there are a few more that are "conditionally" essential for children, since their bodies cannot make enough: arginine, histidine, cysteine, glycine, tyrosine, glutamine, and proline. Provided you give your child a mixture of different protein sources over the course of each day, including whole grains and vegetables, they should have no problem obtaining both essential and conditional amino acids.

VITAMINS AND MINERALS

Consider meeting with your pediatrician and registered dietitian to discuss whether supplementation is necessary:

- **Iron** It's recommended to give all exclusively breastfed babies 1mg per kg (2lb) of body weight a day from four to six months.
- **Vitamin D** Guidance is to supplement with 400 IU of vitamin D for babies who receive only breast milk. Babies fed only formula do not need to supplement since formula is fortified with vitamin D.
- **Iodine** Breast milk and formula provide all requirements. Thereafter, it may be wise to speak to your pediatrician about supplementation.
- **Vitamin B12** There are no quality forms of B12 in a plant-based diet, which is vital for the nervous system, metabolism, and formation of red blood cells. Breast milk will be sufficient only if the mother consumes B12, and formula is fortified already.
- **Choline** Important for babies' brain growth, the main sources of choline are eggs, soy, and cruciferous vegetables.
- **Omega-3** The fatty acid DHA is critical for brain development, but even seaweed, algae, eggs, and fortified foods are unlikely to provide enough, so consider supplements while pregnant and lactating.
- **Calcium** Studies show that calcium, important for growing bones and teeth, can be insufficient in vegan diets. Aim for a variety of fortified plant-based sources: calcium-set tofu, calcium-fortified soy yogurts, baked beans, hummus, and nut butters.

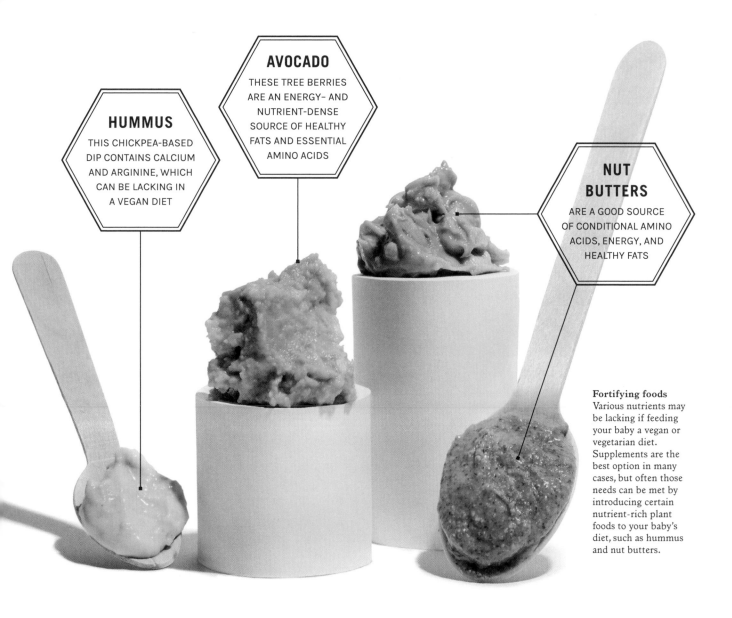

HUMMUS
THIS CHICKPEA-BASED DIP CONTAINS CALCIUM AND ARGININE, WHICH CAN BE LACKING IN A VEGAN DIET

AVOCADO
THESE TREE BERRIES ARE AN ENERGY- AND NUTRIENT-DENSE SOURCE OF HEALTHY FATS AND ESSENTIAL AMINO ACIDS

NUT BUTTERS
ARE A GOOD SOURCE OF CONDITIONAL AMINO ACIDS, ENERGY, AND HEALTHY FATS

Fortifying foods
Various nutrients may be lacking if feeding your baby a vegan or vegetarian diet. Supplements are the best option in many cases, but often those needs can be met by introducing certain nutrient-rich plant foods to your baby's diet, such as hummus and nut butters.

SOURCES OF CONDITIONAL AMINO ACIDS

ARGININE	HISTIDINE	CYSTEINE	TYROSINE	GLUTAMINE	PROLINE
PUMPKIN SEEDS	TOFU	SUNFLOWER SEEDS	MILK	SOYBEANS	BEANS
SOYBEANS	PUMPKIN SEEDS	LENTILS	LENTILS	RED CABBAGE	NUTS
PEANUTS	WHOLE WHEAT PASTA	OATS	PUMPKIN SEEDS	NUTS	SEEDS
CHICKPEAS	NAVY BEANS	CARROTS	WILD RICE	BEANS	
LENTILS					

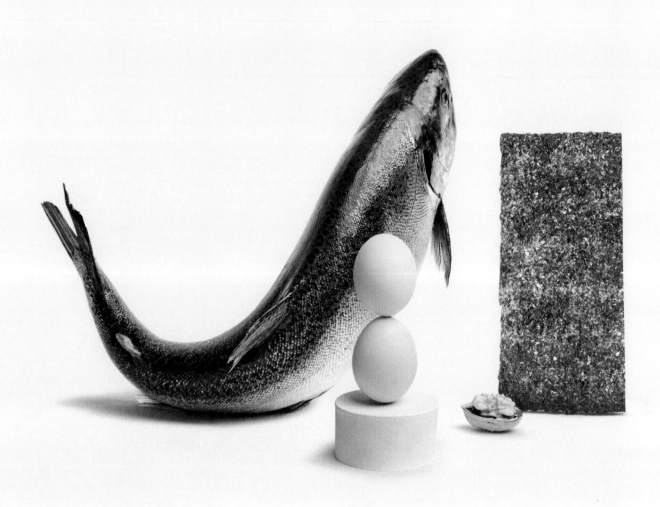

CAN WE EAT TO SUPPORT MENTAL HEALTH?

DOES WHAT I EAT AFFECT MY MOOD?

A healthy diet can do a lot to boost your mood and sense of well-being. In fact, improving what you eat can lead to more positive feelings, clearer thinking, higher energy, and calmer moods.

Research suggests inflammation in the brain is impacted by diet, since short-chain fatty acids produced in the gut have anti-inflammatory properties, and diversity of gut bacteria encourages production of these fatty acids (see pages 48–53). As a result of a poor diet high in salt, saturated fat, and sugars, the hippocampus in the brain decreases in volume and your neurons may be damaged. This in turn can increase the risk of depression, low moods, and poor memory and learning skills. If you aim to follow the Mediterranean diet (see pages 36–41), trials suggest this can act as a treatment for depression and in some cases help prevent it, often proving more impactful than the traditional routes of treatment. To protect your brain, you should also aim to eat more polyphenols, found in foods such as spinach and dark berries like blueberries.

DIET AND THE "HAPPY HORMONE"

Serotonin is a neurotransmitter that helps relay messages from one area of the brain to another and

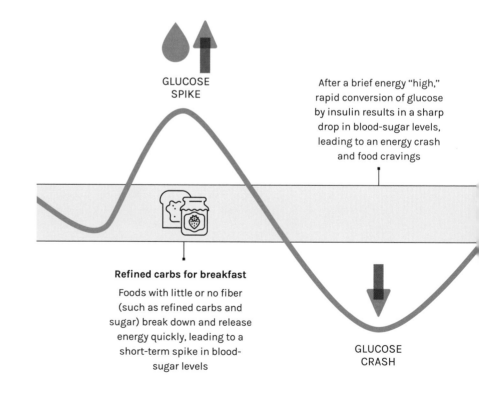

GLUCOSE SPIKE

After a brief energy "high," rapid conversion of glucose by insulin results in a sharp drop in blood-sugar levels, leading to an energy crash and food cravings

GLUCOSE CRASH

Blood sugar highs and lows

When you eat a lot of refined carbs, your pancreas sees a spike in blood glucose levels and releases insulin as quickly as it can to try to catch up. This can result in too much glucose being removed from your blood, causing a blood-sugar crash that can leave you feeling fatigued, irritable, depressed, anxious, and nervous.

Refined carbs for breakfast

Foods with little or no fiber (such as refined carbs and sugar) break down and release energy quickly, leading to a short-term spike in blood-sugar levels

is believed to influence a variety of psychological functions; it's known as the "happy hormone" because of its mood-stabilizing qualities. Gut bacteria manufacture about 95 percent of the body's supply of serotonin and interactions between the gut-brain axis (see pages 48–49), and gut bacteria help you out with many essential functions, such as digestion of nutrients, and may even be implicated in your mental health.

Those of us with low serotonin levels are said to feel better after eating sugar, which is obviously not the healthiest way to lift mood and often leads to binge eating. Instead, you might be able to help serotonin production by consuming plenty of quality carbohydrates and proteins containing the amino acid tryptophan, such as milk or tuna. The research has not yet fully determined whether this dietary change does improve mood, but it may be that not eating enough carbohydrates, for example, in a high-protein/high-fat diet, leads to low moods.

ENERGY AND MOOD

Mood and concentration can be heavily impacted by how dietary choices affect blood-sugar levels. When you eat carbohydrates, your body digests it, converts it into glucose (sugar), and sends the glucose into your blood. Insulin is then produced by the pancreas to convert that glucose into energy.

Your blood-sugar levels are determined by the type of carbohydrates you eat. The wrong type (such as refined carbs and sugar) will send you on a roller-coaster ride that will give you a quick hit of energy, followed by a crash that will leave you feeling low in energy, lacking in concentration, and craving more energy-dense food. This is when you may want to reach for that cookie to give you more sugar. Eating the right type of slow-release carbohydrates, such as whole grains, vegetables, and fruits, however, will keep you safely off the roller coaster, leaving you feeling happier, more focused, and more energetic for longer (see below).

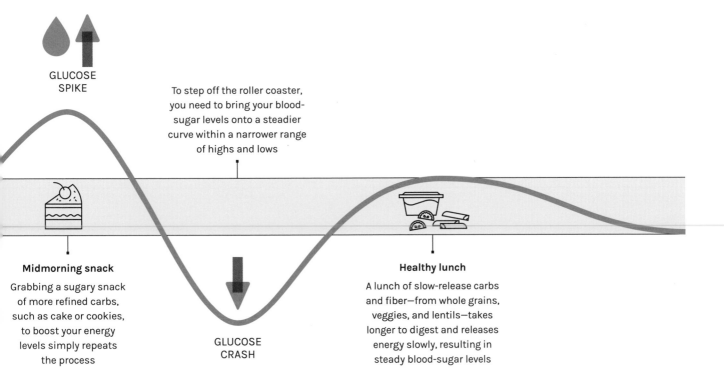

GLUCOSE
SPIKE

To step off the roller coaster, you need to bring your blood-sugar levels onto a steadier curve within a narrower range of highs and lows

Midmorning snack

Grabbing a sugary snack of more refined carbs, such as cake or cookies, to boost your energy levels simply repeats the process

GLUCOSE
CRASH

Healthy lunch

A lunch of slow-release carbs and fiber—from whole grains, veggies, and lentils—takes longer to digest and releases energy slowly, resulting in steady blood-sugar levels

CAN INTUITIVE EATING HELP ME?

Adopting the intuitive-eating approach can help you reconnect with your internal cues, listen to your body, and focus on health instead of weight.

Many people think intuitive eating (IE) is an all-or-nothing approach (much like a diet), but IE is a nondiet approach that helps individuals heal from chronic dieting. It encourages you to ditch food rules, respect your body, and actually enjoy food again.

CHOOSING THE CHOCOLATE

When you are constantly dieting, food choices often come with little enjoyment and a side of guilt, as you choose what you think you should be eating. However, this can often backfire. For example, you crave some chocolate, but you think, "It's not healthy," so you opt for a low-calorie snack instead. You feel unsatisfied after eating this snack, so you search for something else … and so the pattern continues. If you had listened to your body and eaten the chocolate, you likely would have satisfied your stomach and not needed to overeat.

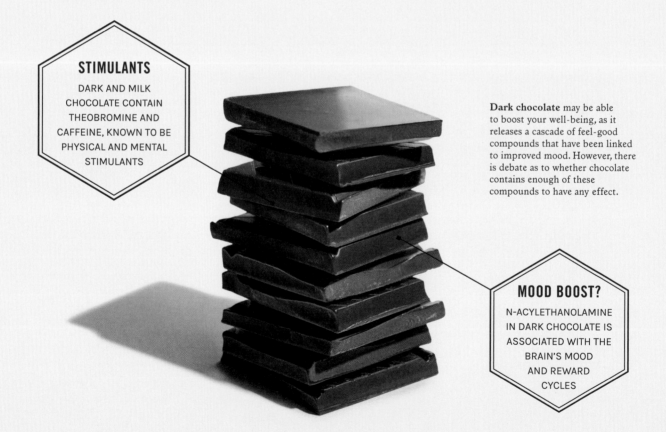

STIMULANTS
DARK AND MILK CHOCOLATE CONTAIN THEOBROMINE AND CAFFEINE, KNOWN TO BE PHYSICAL AND MENTAL STIMULANTS

Dark chocolate may be able to boost your well-being, as it releases a cascade of feel-good compounds that have been linked to improved mood. However, there is debate as to whether chocolate contains enough of these compounds to have any effect.

MOOD BOOST?
N-ACYLETHANOLAMINE IN DARK CHOCOLATE IS ASSOCIATED WITH THE BRAIN'S MOOD AND REWARD CYCLES

THE INTUITIVE EATING APPROACH IS MADE UP OF 10 PRINCIPLES:

1.
REJECT THE DIET MENTALITY

Address your food rules, which can be influenced by external factors like diets and the media. If you have a history of disordered eating, they will take time to undo.

2.
HONOR HUNGER

You are "allowed" to be hungry. Hunger means our body's signals are working, but diets often require us to ignore them. Hunger cues include feeling light-headed, irritable, or low on energy.

3.
MAKE PEACE WITH FOOD

Give yourself permission to eat. This doesn't mean always binging on unhealthy foods. By allowing all foods, "forbidden" loses its appeal, and you strike a balance.

4.
CHALLENGE THE FOOD POLICE

Call out the voice in your head that tries to dictate your food choices based on calorie content or "health.'. Think more rationally around food.

5.
RESPECT FULLNESS

There is a difference between feeling full and feeling satisfied. Check in with yourself as you are eating. Are you satisfied or getting full? Mindful eating might be helpful here (see pages 206-207).

6.
DISCOVER THE SATISFACTION FACTOR

To eat less and feel more fulfilled, choose delicious foods you really want and will satisfy. Prioritize a few meals a week to focus on positive eating, to begin with.

7.
DISASSOCIATE FEELINGS FROM FOOD

When comfort eating becomes your only coping mechanism, it can be problematic. Try to find other ways to comfort—taking a bath, reading a book, going for a walk.

8.
ACCEPT BODY DIVERSITY

We come in all different shapes and sizes and should not sacrifice health to try to change our genes. Consider psychological support if you struggle with body image.

9.
EXERCISE—FEEL THE DIFFERENCE

Movement is good for physical and mental health and should feel good. Explore different forms of movement that make you feel energized—and ditch the tracking devices .

10.
TAKE NUTRITION GENTLY

You must first explore your relationship with food and then consider the basics of nutrition. It is important to eat for well-being as well as enjoyment.

CAN MINDFUL EATING HELP ME?

Too often, eating is something to get done quickly while we multitask.
But if we take the time to develop a mindful approach to eating,
our relationship with food can drastically improve.

Whenever we eat or drink, we have the opportunity to focus on the moment. Unfortunately, many of us don't do this; instead, we eat while talking on the phone or working on the computer, barely noticing the taste or the amount of food we are consuming. With mindful eating, we direct our full awareness to the sensations, thoughts, and emotions that arise as we eat, without criticism or judgment. We notice the colors, shapes, fragrances, flavors, textures, and even sounds of our food. A big movement toward mindful eating has begun, suggesting that slower and more thoughtful eating can help combat weight problems and poor food choices.

AM I EATING MINDFULLY?

Do you feel in control of the decisions you make around food every day? When you go to the movies, are you aware of how much popcorn you are eating, or are you so distracted by the movie that you finish off the whole bucket, without really tasting it? Being aware of how you eat is key. Only then can you move forward and rebuild your relationship with food. We have taste buds for a reason, and feeling full is a natural sensation, so allow yourself to enjoy your food. This is the first step to eating mindfully.

MAKING CHANGES

Key to mindful eating is recognizing the mindless eating habits that we all engage in at some time or other. Look at the list opposite, identify which habits you regularly fall into, and develop strategies to change them. Be conscious of what, when, and how you eat, and take the time to appreciate your food and enjoy the experience as often as you can.

NO PORTION CONTROL
Piling the plate high
when you're hungry is easy to do. Try weighing ingredients before you cook and sticking to sensible portion sizes.

NIGHTTIME SNACKING
Avoid skipping meals
and make sure you eat enough during the day to avoid nighttime hunger pangs that interrupt your sleep.

USING TECHNOLOGY
at mealtimes
Watching television or scrolling on your phone while eating will distract you from your food. Try to put your phone in another room and turn off the TV during mealtimes.

MOODY EATER
when angry, bored, tired, or stressed
Most people comfort eat sometimes, but if you do this often, try to find other ways to boost your mood, such as exercising, taking a bath, or journaling.

PICKING ON FOOD

throughout the day

Grazing all day on snacks will likely lead to short-term energy spikes followed by blood-sugar crashes (see pages 202–203). Try eating substantial meals with complex carbohydrates for a slower release of energy.

EATING ON THE COUCH

instead of at the table

The couch is a place to lounge and relax. Eating at the table will encourage a better posture for eating and greater attention to your food.

EATING ON THE GO

When you're dashing

from place to place, eating becomes an expedient rather than a priority. Try to stop, even for five minutes, to savor your food.

EATING WHATEVER

is in the office that day at your desk

Sometimes convenience wins, but try to deliberately choose food you want to eat, and step away from your desk and any other distractions to enjoy it.

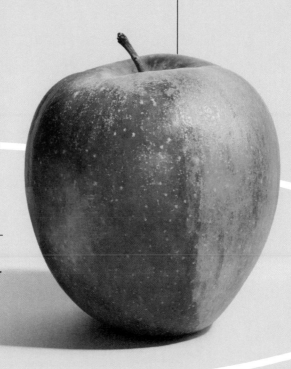

Mindless eating habits to guard against

Ask yourself how often you engage in these mindless eating habits and whether you can change your behavior. You might not be able to avoid all of them all the time, but being aware of them means you change the areas you choose to.

EATING OVERLY PROCESSED FOODS

Processed and packaged

foods have all sorts of hidden ingredients in them, many of them unhealthy. Try cooking from scratch as often as you can, so you know what's going into your food.

WEEKEND EATER

You're good all week, then it goes out the window on the weekend

Give yourself permission to eat more freely all the time, rather than being restrictive during the week and binge eating on the weekend.

NOT CHEWING FOOD

Shoveling down food

without chewing makes it harder for the body to digest and will leave you feeling unsatisfied and likely to overeat. Try to allow sufficient time to enjoy your meal or snack, and eat slowly.

SKIPPING BREAKFAST

This can seem like a quick fix

if you're in a hurry or looking to cut down on food intake, but taking time for a healthy breakfast will set you up for the day with slow-release energy and prevent you from overeating at lunch.

The binge-restrict cycle

Restricting unhealthy foods may seem like the right thing to do, but it can kick-start a pattern of bingeing.

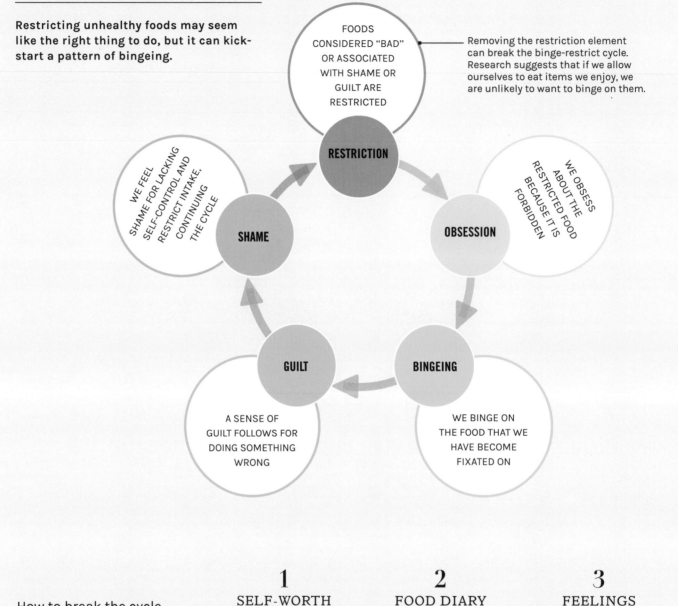

FOODS CONSIDERED "BAD" OR ASSOCIATED WITH SHAME OR GUILT ARE RESTRICTED

Removing the restriction element can break the binge-restrict cycle. Research suggests that if we allow ourselves to eat items we enjoy, we are unlikely to want to binge on them.

RESTRICTION

WE FEEL SHAME FOR LACKING SELF-CONTROL AND RESTRICT INTAKE, CONTINUING THE CYCLE

SHAME

OBSESSION

WE OBSESS ABOUT THE RESTRICTED FOOD BECAUSE IT IS FORBIDDEN

GUILT

BINGEING

A SENSE OF GUILT FOLLOWS FOR DOING SOMETHING WRONG

WE BINGE ON THE FOOD THAT WE HAVE BECOME FIXATED ON

How to break the cycle

The binge-restrict cycle can happen to anybody, not just those with eating disorders. If you ever find yourself stuck in the binge-restrict cycle, think about the following:

1 SELF-WORTH

Be prepared to work on yourself.

Analyze your expectations and values and learn to grow your self-worth and self-esteem. Seek the help of a professional therapist if necessary.

2 FOOD DIARY

Work on a food–mood diary.

See pages 96–97. Eat three balanced meals a day and two to three snacks; enough to maintain your body weight—you need to get out of the binge-restrict cycle before trying to lose weight.

3 FEELINGS

Understand your feelings.

What is your eating style? Are there a lot of rules? Feelings of guilt or sadness? How do you feel if you break one of your rules, and how do you respond?

HOW CAN I STOP BINGE EATING?

Binge eating is often explained as eating when we're not hungry or overeating to provide a temporary distraction from something painful. But the relationship between food and mood goes far beyond that specific moment.

Emotional eating is often a way of compensating for a lack of coping skills. And for some, this pattern can become a compulsion. It's important to note that binge-eating disorder is a serious mental illness where people who eat large quantities of food can feel like they are out of control, which can be incredibly distressing. Binges can leave the individual feeling disconnected from what they're doing during a binge. They can even forget what they have eaten afterward.

AM I BINGE EATING?

Everyone is an emotional eater to some degree. Stress, boredom, anxiety, or sleep-deprivation can make us want to eat more of different foods (or not eat). The problem occurs when our emotions rule how we eat. If we overeat in response to something difficult or painful, we can get caught in the binge-restrict cycle (see left). A binge is followed by guilt, even shame and embarrassment, which can cause an individual to restrict their food intake to compensate. Restriction triggers obsessive thoughts of food and so the cycle begins again. If you can spend time developing new coping strategies for emotional issues, it may help you get to the core of what is really going on and beat the binge-restrict cycle.

If you believe you're suffering from any form of disordered eating, you should seek professional help at the earliest opportunity. Your doctor should be your first point of contact as they can refer you to a qualified health professional. Alternatively, seek support from a registered therapist.

4	5	6
TRIGGERS	NEGATIVE THOUGHTS	KINDNESS

Identify your triggers.

See whether you can recognize yourself in any of the common binge eating triggers below and think about how these states might affect you throughout your day: Anger | Anxiety | Worry | Fear Depression | Negativity | Boredom Guilt | Shame

Challenge negative thoughts.

Consider naming that inner critic inside your head. You may be surprised to find that you are bullying yourself— a sign that some self-soothing is required.

Be kind to yourself.

Remember that your body needs food for fuel. If your body is receiving the nutrition it needs, you are less likely to suffer from ill health. You deserve to eat and enjoy food.

AM I SUFFERING FROM DISORDERED EATING?

An eating disorder is a complex mental illness and is often deeply misunderstood. Anyone, of any gender, age, ethnicity, shape, and size, can get one—they do not discriminate.

A healthy relationship with food enables you to eat a variety of foods in a flexible and spontaneous way. This relationship can look different to us all, but ultimately it means that food does not interfere with your life and you do not have to live by certain dietary rules, such as only eating carbohydrates if you have exercised that day.

WHAT IS DISORDERED EATING?

People with eating disorders use disordered eating as a way of coping with difficult situations or feelings. This behavior can include limiting food intake; eating very large quantities of food at once; getting rid of eaten food through unhealthy means (e.g., vomiting, misusing laxatives, fasting, or exercising excessively); or a combination of these.

There's no single cause, and sufferers might not have all the symptoms of any one eating disorder. Perhaps the most commonly recognized is anorexia nervosa, but you don't have to be underweight to have anorexia. And you can develop symptoms of one eating disorder that then change over time and transform into another; for example, symptoms of anorexia can develop into a diagnosis for bulimia. Stereotypes about those who get eating disorders might make them even harder to spot among older people, men and boys, and ethnic and cultural minority groups. Many people are diagnosed with "other specified feeding or eating disorder" (OSFED), which means their symptoms don't exactly match what doctors check for to diagnose binge-eating disorder, anorexia, or bulimia, but that doesn't mean that it's not still very serious.

Recognizing the symptoms

EATING DISORDERS MANIFEST DIFFERENTLY FROM PERSON TO PERSON, WHICH CAN MAKE THEM TRICKY TO SPOT. HERE ARE SOME SIGNS TO LOOK OUT FOR:

BEHAVIORAL SIGNS

- Spending a lot of time worrying about your weight and body shape
- Avoiding socializing when you think food will be involved
- Eating very little food
- Making yourself vomit or taking laxatives after you eat
- Exercising too much
- Having very strict habits or routines around food
- Changes in your mood, such as being withdrawn, anxious, or depressed

PHYSICAL SIGNS

- Feeling cold, tired, or dizzy
- Pains, tingling, or numbness in your arms and legs (poor circulation)
- Racing heartbeat, fainting, or feeling faint
- Problems with your digestion, such as bloating, constipation, or diarrhea
- Your weight being very high or very low for someone of your age and height
- Not getting your period or other delayed signs of puberty

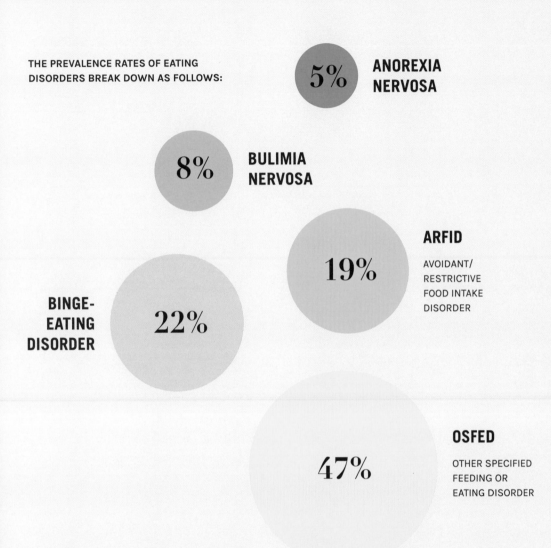

THE PREVALENCE RATES OF EATING DISORDERS BREAK DOWN AS FOLLOWS:

5% ANOREXIA NERVOSA

8% BULIMIA NERVOSA

19% ARFID
AVOIDANT/ RESTRICTIVE FOOD INTAKE DISORDER

BINGE-EATING DISORDER **22%**

47% OSFED
OTHER SPECIFIED FEEDING OR EATING DISORDER

EATING DISORDERS AFFECT AT LEAST **9%** OF THE POPULATION WORLDWIDE

AROUND **70 million** PEOPLE INTERNATIONALLY LIVE WITH EATING DISORDERS

AROUND **9%** OF THE U.S. POPULATION WILL SUFFER AN EATING DISORDER DURING THEIR LIFE

SOME **28.8 million** PEOPLE

OF WHOM **1/3** ARE MALE

LESS THAN **6%** OF PEOPLE DIAGNOSED WITH EATING DISORDERS ARE MEDICALLY UNDERWEIGHT

WHAT HELP CAN I GET?

If you suspect you have an eating disorder, try to see your primary care physician (PCP) right away—the sooner, the better. Ask for a double appointment to give you time to talk. You can bring a support person, though some PCPs may ask to speak to you alone for some of the time. Give as much information as possible; try noting symptoms and concerns ahead of time. Your PCP should refer you to a specialist who can assess your needs and develop a plan for treatment.

Sometimes people think their eating disorder isn't serious enough and don't want to waste people's time; or they feel guilty, ashamed, or embarrassed. PCPs don't specialize in eating disorders and may harbor misconceptions. Look for local support groups that can help you get connected to help. If a referral to a specialist isn't the result of your appointment, you have the right to ask to see a different PCP. Don't be daunted and don't give up; you deserve treatment, and research suggests recovery is possible at any time.

INDEX

ACKNOWLEDGMENTS

BIBLIOGRAPHY

To access a comprehensive list of source materials, studies, and research supporting the information in this book, please visit: **www.dk.com/science-of-nutrition-biblio**

AUTHOR'S ACKNOWLEDGMENTS

Although writing a few words will never repay the faith so many people have shown in me, I hope it goes some way to telling them how forever grateful I am.

Of course, thank you to everyone at DK for inviting me on such an inspiring project. It's an honor to work with such a dedicated publisher that shares my passion for evidence-based advice. It has been a real pleasure to work with you, Alastair, Katie, and Dawn. The extraordinary contribution of editors Andrea, Holly, Salima, and Megan in refining my work deserves an immense thanks. It must also be said, the truly outstanding quality of this book is its design, with special thanks to Alison for being so innovative.

It is my earliest teachers, who fostered such a respect and passion for science, without whom I would not be who I am or doing what I do. In particular, I would like to thank Dr. Sue Reeves, Kirsty Cotton, and The University of Roehampton, all instrumental in launching my nutrition career.

Thanks to all those who took the time out of their busy schedules to read and critically review every page; my mentor Jennifer Low, my amazing gut health dietitian Kaitlin Colucci, my sports nutritionist Faye Townsend, intuitive eating nutritionist Sophie Bertrand, and medical review by Dr. P.—your stamp of approval means so much more knowing how close a friend you are to me.

To my remarkable Rhitrition team: Bea, Jen, Kaitlin, Faye, Sophie, Sarah, Caff, Hala, Katie, and Victoria. The only thing that makes me prouder than all the good we've done together is the thought of all the remarkable things you'll achieve from here.

I also want to thank my husband and son, you bring with you endless joy and love. You have been there for me through the toughest of pandemic times. Juggling motherhood and business in lockdown seemed impossible, but you help me believe that I can achieve anything I set my mind to and make me an infinitely better person.

Last but not least, I would like to thank all of you out there. Whether by following me @Rhitrition, buying a book, or seeing me in clinic, you are showing how much you value science. Amidst a confusing postpandemic time, this feels more important now than ever, I know you have all been through hardships. That's also why I leave writing this book even more optimistic about our health than I was when I started. Because I know this book will not only help so many people; it will inspire more to believe you can make a difference to your health and that of the planet, too, knowing nutrition is a science.

PUBLISHER'S ACKNOWLEDGMENTS

Dorling Kindersley would like to thank Megan Lea for editorial assistance; Mandy Earey for design assistance; Ginger Hultin for consulting; Marie Lorimer for indexing; Pankaj Sharma and Vikram Singh for reprographic work; Hayley Dodd for food styling; and Steve Crozier for image retouching.

ABOUT THE AUTHOR

Rhiannon Lambert is one of the UK's leading nutritionists, a best-selling author and chart-topping podcast host.

In 2016 she founded Rhitrition, a renowned Harley Street clinic, which specializes in weight management, sports nutrition, eating disorders, and pre- and post-natal nutrition. Its highly qualified, professional team of registered nutritionists, registered dietitians, and chartered psychologists work with individuals to transform their lives.

As an evidence-based practitioner, Rhiannon is committed to the benefits of a scientific approach to nutrition.

She has worked as a consultant to many well-known food brands including Deliveroo, Wagamana, Alpro, Yeo Valley, and Little Freddie, refining their menus, product ranges, and cooking methodology. Rhiannon has also advised on nutrition and wellbeing at Six Senses, Four Seasons Hotels & Resorts, Amazon, Microsoft, Samsung, and Coty.

In 2017, Rhiannon published her first book, the best-selling *Re-Nourish: A Simple Way To Eat Well*, part handbook, part cookbook, in which she shares her food philosophy to lay the foundations for a happy, healthy relationship with eating. She followed this up with *Top Of Your Game: Eating For Mind & Body*, co-written with world snooker champion, Ronnie O'Sullivan.

Rhiannon also has her own food supplements company, RhiNourish. A healthy, balanced diet should provide all the nutrients your body needs but, sometimes, for all sorts of reasons, it falls short. RhiNourish's innovative approach uses Rhiannon's evidence-based, scientifically sound formulas to produce supplements for the vitamins and minerals lacking in many diets.

Rhiannon hosts the top-rated "Food for Thought" podcast which gives listeners practical, evidence-based advice on how to achieve a healthier lifestyle. With more than five million downloads since 2018, it is firmly established as one of the UK's most popular health podcasts.

Registered with the Association for Nutrition, Rhiannon obtained a first-class degree in Nutrition and Health, a Master's degree in Obesity, Risks, and Prevention, and diplomas in sports nutrition, and in pre- and post-natal nutrition. She is a Master Practitioner in Eating Disorders, accredited by The British Psychological Society, and a Level 3 Personal Trainer.

Follow Rhiannon on Instagram, Twitter, Facebook, and YouTube at @Rhitrition and visit Rhitrition.com